JUST BENEATH THE SURFACE

NICOLE BOAND, RN, DC

COPYRIGHT © 1994 BY NICOLE BOAND

All rights reserved. No part of this book may be reproduced or transmitted in any form or by any means, graphic, electronic, or mechanical, including photocopying, recording, or any information storage or retrieval system, for sale, without written permission from the author, except for brief quotations included in a review.

Edited by Joseph Jaeger

Cover Design by Thomas Taylor of Thomcatt Graphics

Vista Publishing, Inc.
473 Broadway
Long Branch, New Jersey 07740
(908) 229-6500

This publication is designed for the reading pleasure of the general public. The story depicts the thoughts and feelings of the author and are based on her experiences. The opinions are that of the author.

Printed and bound in the United States of America.

First Edition

ISBN: 1-880254-14-X
Library of Congress Catalog Card Number 93-61854

U.S.A. Price $12.95
Canada Price $18.95

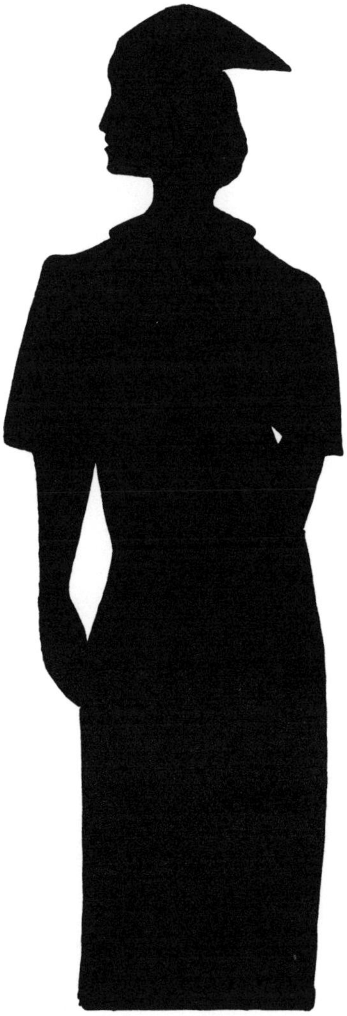

for

Catherine Jaynne

and

Harry Boand

About the Author

Nicole Boand received a BA in psychology from the University of Southern California and earned her diploma in nursing from the Los Angeles County School of Nursing, located at the LAC-USC Medical Center. After working as an R.N. for several years she returned to school and earned a Doctor of Chiropractic degree from Cleveland Chiropractic College in 1986. **Just Beneath the Surface** is her first book.

Dr. Boand is currently living on the Monterey Peninsula with her husband Larry Dalton who holds the Harold Moulton endowed professorship of chemistry and is Co-director of the Loker Hydrocarbon Research Institute at USC. Together they have traveled extensively throughout the world. When not traveling she spends her time writing, painting, and galloping her horse along the ocean. Her art work is currently being sold in Carmel California and Vail Colorado.

Contents

Forward

1/	Welcome to County	1
2/	County Life Begins, Real Life Ends	5
3/	Breakfast, Lunch, and Dinner, For Fifteen Dollars A Month	7
4/	Mother Merlin Leads The Way	17
5/	Co-Ed Volleyball	23
6/	The Art of Nursing	28
7/	Party Manners	35
8/	Angel In White	39
9/	This Is Just A Friendship, and Other Sweet Lies I Have Told Myself	42
10/	This Is Just A Friendship, But I Think I'll Pack Some Birth Control	44
11/	Capping	50
12/	The Troll Under The Bridge	57
13/	It Only Takes A Five To Pass	61
14/	The Queen Of Psychosocial Nursing	66
15/	Lost In The Joy Of Romance	73
16/	The Light Of Day	78
17/	"I Don't Know Nothin' Bout Birthin' Babies."	82
18/	A Play Siren Searches For A Pal	94
19/	Lessons In Living	102
20/	Romance Redeux	108

Contents Continued:

21/ "You Must Conceptualize"	117
22/ The Girls Go Traveling	129
23/ Macho Nursing	133
24/ Mindless Movement	144
25/ Tending The Garden	153
26/ After Hours	163
27/ Rites Of Passage	171
28/ Into The Night	176
29/ Finishing Touches	180
30/ Pomp and Circumstance	192 |//
Afterward	

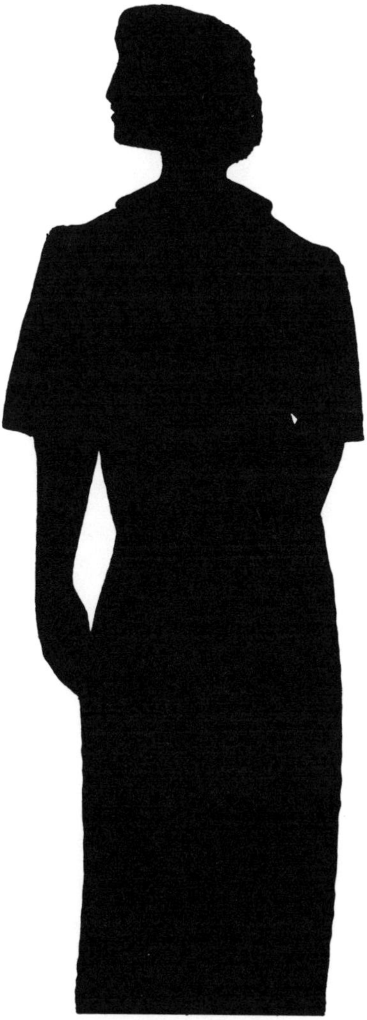

Forward

      I wrote this book because nursing is not what you see on the surface of the man or woman in white at the hospital bedside. It has to do with what goes on between patients and nurses, doctors and nurses, and among the nurses themselves. The art of delivering health care, when done well, is an act of heart and mind. The use of only one of these resources is not sufficient to get the job done properly.

      The complexities of what faced us as students at County went beyond learning the physical tasks of nursing. We were confronted with the difficulties of delivering health care to vast numbers of immigrants who spoke no English, indigent homeless patients, and patients from diverse cultural backgrounds and belief systems. Our instructors attempted to teach us the magic of delivering health care on a shoestring budget, while maintaining the dignity of our patients.

      This book follows the transformation of myself and my classmates from struggling nursing students to practicing professionals. This journey, by its very nature, is one of self discovery.

Chapter One

Welcome to County

An empty dorm room is depressing, and the furnishings make the Shaker's homes look extravagant. I had been married and divorced, owned my own home and sold it in the dissolution of the marriage. Standing in this room felt overwhelmingly regressive to me. Eight years of living and I was back at the level of a college freshman.

The room was long and narrow, with a sink and closet at one end, and a window at the other. All the rooms were painted in a variety of pastel shades; mine was institutional yellow. It could have been worse: some people got aqua. While the steel frame twin bed pushed against the wall was the most depressing, it was the sheets that made it unbearable. Included in the monthly dorm fee of forty dollars was linen service. I acknowledge this is a wonderful bargain. But the towels and sheets were the same ones that were used in the hospital. They were stiff, scratchy, and smelled strongly of disinfectant.

There are some stains that do not come out, no matter how strong the detergent. Blood, betadine (surgical scrub soap), and ball point pen last forever. Occasionally interns have the nasty habit of writing their patient's vital signs in ink on the bed sheets. This includes heart rate, blood pressure, respirations, and temperature. I assume this mostly went on with patients who were in a coma and couldn't be offended by this personal data scrawled next to their pillow. My stomach would sink as I crawled into bed on sheets with someone's failing heart rate permanently inscribed on them. I was determined to find an apartment immediately.

I was twenty-six and considered myself pretty old to be embarking on a nursing career. Conflicting images of blossoming Mother Theresas and student nurses romping through the hospital hallways with their panties showing troubled me. Within every stereotype there are variations; I was prepared to match none of them. I expected to spend the next two years as something of an aloof older alien among fresh young faces.

County's School of Nursing frightened me for many reasons. It is an enormous inner city teaching hospital, located in one of the most dangerous areas of Los Angeles. County's patients are not just sick, they are desperately ill or dying. The school's reputation for producing exceptionally well trained nurses was both alluring and intimidating. It was appealing to be affiliated with the best, but it also meant the program would be emotionally and academically demanding. Anxiety had been building up in me for weeks by the time I climbed the school's front steps.

The nursing dorm lobby was filled with our class of over a hundred new students. The students presented a more varied picture than I had expected. This was not a group of twenty year old girls. My classmates varied in age from nineteen to nearly fifty. Almost one third of our class was over twenty-five and about fifteen of our members were men.

Pressing in on the crowd from above was a myriad of homemade posters. They hung suspended from the ceiling by long chains made of paper clips. Waiting in line to register gave me time to study these posters. Their artistic quality ranged from elementary to high school election posters. With varying degrees of neatness, wide felt tip markers spelled out the names of individual students in large block letters. One hanging inches from my nose announced, "Karen Kaplin R.N., Yeah We Made It!" A collage of photos filled up the space under the bright red letters. The same smiling plump brunette could be found somewhere in each photo. There were shots of Karen drinking beer with her buddies, standing with people who looked like her parents, and Karen holding someone's baby.

Studying these strange posters made the time in line pass more quickly. I couldn't imagine myself making and displaying anything so juvenile and self-congratulatory. The woman in front of me spoke my thoughts out loud. "What is with all this weird shit hanging around?"

My first life long friend at County had just spoken. Her imperious demeanor was accentuated by her height. At five feet ten she had two very impressive inches on me. She held herself erect, her chin tilted up, her dark eyes glancing down her nose. I agreed with her the posters were strange. She countered by extending her hand, "My name is Evelyn."

Evelyn then introduced me to the others she had collected around her. She had just met these people, but they already had the cohesive presence of a group. There was Gregory who would turn nineteen in three days, but could easily pass for thirty. If you included the top of his Afro he looked about six foot six, and gorgeous. Susan was next; she appeared to be about my age. She had a blasé, sophisticated presentation. Finally there was Ann, short, blond, and bubbly. I became the fifth member of Evelyn's clique.

We had made our way through the final line of the morning. Upon reaching the end of this line we were required to hand over a check or money order. We each received the key to a dorm room in exchange. The majority of students who attended County General School of Nursing lived in the dorms. I had recently returned to the area and had expectations of finding a cozy, charming, inexpensive apartment in Pasadena. But as a new student, I had been assigned to the dorm. This was fine. I needed a place to leave my luggage and stuff until I found my apartment.

Upon receiving our keys everyone took off upstairs to examine the rooms. Cubicles was a better word, or possibly cells. I'm not sure of the size, maybe fifteen by twelve feet, whatever. A small bathroom with a toilet and a stall shower joined two rooms together, creating a "suite." This provided one with a "suite mate." Despite the surroundings, there was a level of care and consideration underlying certain aspects of life at County. A woman in admissions had taken the time to match up suite mates, using her own judgment about who belonged with whom.

Susan and I were assigned as suite mates. We were nearly a perfect match. She was twenty-seven and had a bachelor's degree in sociology. My bachelor's was in psychology. Our universities were cross-town rivals. We were also physically matched, both tall and slim. Some people might have called us thin, but these are people who aren't slim and don't know the difference.

I recall having a couple of days available to me after that initial day of registration before classes and day to day life at County actually began. I camped out at the apartment of my friend Jeff. He was one of my best friends and we had great sex together. We thought we were pulling off the ultimate friendship. We were going to avoid the traps of romance and monogamy.

The days at Jeff's place were spent in a search for the perfect apartment and finally any affordable living space. I had set my lower limits; neighborhoods requiring burglar bars were definitely the cut off point. I came to understand that places which do not have bars on the windows cost about two hundred dollars a month more than I could afford. Finally, I was shown a dirty studio apartment, about six cubic feet larger than the dorm room at County. This place did have a bar-size refrigerator and a built-in hot plate and only cost a hundred dollars a month more than I could afford.

I spent a night in tears, and had a long phone call with my father, making sure I had an accurate picture of my financial situation. I did. He offered me a loan to help with my rent. I had just enough monthly income from an investment to live in the nursing school dorm and pay my tuition without working. My fear of being in debt was greater than my disgust at the dorms. My room on the seventh floor was my home for the next two years.

I have strong nesting instincts. I am one of those people who could make a cardboard box feel a little bit homey. After about two weeks of retrieving pieces of furniture stored with friends and family, and buying a forty dollar rug, my room felt enough like a home to comfort me. I placed an oval table against the wall. This was for my bird, Chrome. Birds were one of the only pets we were allowed to have at County; mine was a cockatiel named after Aldous Huxley's novel **Chrome Yellow**. He turned out to be a she, and her head never did turn yellow, and therefore her name became Chromina. She had a cage and a play pen, but she preferred to sit under my desk, eating and pooping on my files. Mostly, Chrome played hide and seek whenever I tried to find her. The room was completed after I sneaked my waterbed frame up the back stairs of the dorm. Pushed into the corner of the room, the double bed was within arm's reach of the telephone. My attitude improved immensely upon removal of the twin bed. County sheets were relegated to mopping up very large spills.

The first two weeks at County were one long blurring assault on my senses. I come from an upper middle class, white bread kind of background. My mother was actually prettier than Donna Reed or June Cleaver, and just as loving and kind. Nobody comes through childhood scar free. My scars were of the internal sort caused by a turmoil of emotions. But my experiences had taken place in clean, comfortable surroundings. People were healthy, voices were seldom raised, emotions were moderated, and politeness was greatly valued.

I had no idea why I had this overwhelming compulsion to put myself through two years of living, eating, and working in a county hospital. It was absolutely worse than my worst fantasy. The sights, smells, and sounds were more odious than one can possibly imagine unless you have experienced them. I had already heard rumors of the types of jobs we would be required to do. Putting tubes down peoples' noses and up their genitals, changing wound dressings, and suctioning respirators. Each piece of news was increasingly horrifying. But I didn't turn and run away. I didn't even make a graceful exit with my head held high, saying this was not the place for me.

I stayed and faced County, one day at a time. I decided to rush my dragons, eyes closed, terrified, and ferocious, determined to survive. It was all just beneath the surface. My best guess is that the world saw a tall, pretty young woman, who appeared bright, stand-offish, and had an air of superiority. My strengths are also my traps. I am an excellent facade builder. Throughout my life as a terrified dragon slayer, I have intimidated and repelled many.

Chapter Two

County Life Begins - Real Life Ends

Certain faces from that first day of orientation are frozen in my memory forever. Evelyn's is such a face. I loved Evelyn from the moment I saw her: tall, beautiful and strong. Evelyn had the best "don't fuck with me" attitude of any woman I'd known. She did it with grace, style, and power. Like magnets we had strong sides that attracted and strong sides that repelled. Our friendship has remained a mix of hot and cold with an underlying bond of love.

I can't imagine how we appeared to other people. We were a black and white version of the same facade. But I always felt Evelyn did it better; possibly because I never knew her panic. I only felt my own. There is an understanding I have found among women who are external towers of strength and control. We gravitate towards each other. We love and admire each other's capabilities. We have a sense of knowing one another. But we do not pick, we do not probe, we accept each other's explanations and rationalizations. With an unspoken self-knowledge, we respect the delicate balance of a facade. Even the builder does not always know which bricks can be safely removed.

My suite mate Susan formed the third corner of our triangle. Some trios are awkward, some are so perfectly balanced that they cannot stand with just two. Our trio was a series of two person relationships that managed to all blend fairly smoothly. We shared different parts of our characters with different people.

Susan and I immediately checked out each other's libraries and were delighted. One rarely comes across another Jane Austen fan; she had all of Austen's novels. Looking back on people I have loved, I can always remember what I received from them. I rarely know what I gave to them. I know that Susan introduced me to science fiction, and to one of my all-time favorite books, ***Six of One,*** by Rita Mae Brown.

Susan was political and a radical. I am rather apolitical and believe strongly in personal responsibility. We would explain to each other how we viewed the world, and why our own view was more rational (mine), or humane (hers). We could get pretty heated in these discussions. There was no win or lose; we were engaging in mental gymnastics.

I don't remember Evelyn ever involved in these discussions. She and I rarely exchanged books; we exchanged "Vogue" and "Cosmopolitan." Both Evelyn and I have a controlled passion for clothing that is daring or different. If a piece is slightly alarming, we are sure to be intrigued. Susan's closet, in contrast, was quite stark. Her room was also somewhat bare; she didn't seem to need as many things around her.

Evelyn and Susan had a strong friendship of their own, one that did not involve me. I think it was centered on men. I related to men differently than Evelyn or Susan. I believe we each had our own personal craziness when it came to men; theirs just happened to match a little better. But we all kept one another pretty well informed on the intimate details of our sex lives. It amazes me how free I can be with information on my sex life, and how guarded I am on the workings of my heart.

It is not yet time to talk about men. They were present - the fourth floor of the dorms was the men's floor. But my first encounters with County were so absorbing that it gave my almost constant attraction to men a brief respite (a week or two). During those first days I was aware of the men around me but was too busy to deal with them.

Chapter Three

Breakfast, Lunch and Dinner for Fifteen Dollars a Month

County Hospital is actually made up of four hospitals. The grounds are approximately four miles long and two and one-half miles wide. It is a city within a city. County even has its own division of the sheriff's department. Underground there is another smaller city, containing kitchens, bakeries, laundries, maintenance, generators, etc., all connected by a series of tunnels large enough for small trucks to roll through. It's possible to travel anywhere in the County complex underground, if you are brave enough. At the time I attended County, it was the largest medical complex in the world.

Numbers make very little difference to me in the long run. What mattered was that County was immense. Every day more people were fed at County than live in many towns in the U. S. Just to bake enough bread for this many people is amazing. You can't also expect it to be good.

Three meals a day, seven days a week, for fifteen dollars a month - this is a bargain. The food is all prepared and waiting for you. You just walk in, line up, show your meal card and eat it. Breakfast and dinner were served in the doctors' cafeteria, lunch was in the student nurses' cafeteria. The two were about a hundred yards apart on the first floor of the main hospital.

County doesn't have some very sick patients - all County patients are very sick. County doesn't have some exhausted doctors - all County doctors are exhausted. So to say the cafeterias are on the first floor of the main hospital, is to say they are entrenched in the very center of this mass of souls. Souls who are fighting for their lives, souls who are battling the great nemesis of disease in mankind, and souls who are just paid to work here.

Breakfast service started at six AM on weekdays. The dorm was located off to the side of the main hospital and across the street from the psychiatric hospital. The walk to the cafeteria began pleasantly enough, down my hall to the elevator, down the elevator to the dorm lobby, and out the back door of the lobby to the stairs.

The cement stair led up to a walkway, leading to a side entrance of the main hospital, affectionately known to Countyites as Unit One. I usually enjoyed the walk up these stairs. There were ferns and trees on either side. I felt like I was in a large diorama at Disneyland. I shared this concept with others, but nobody seemed to grasp the connection like I did. The foliage here looked like a prehistoric setting; I always kept watch for dinosaurs.

I had been living by the shore of a beautiful lake in Oregon before coming to County. This cement walk through the palm trees and ferns was as close to nature as I got. One evening, soon after my arrival, I heard a rustling sound in the ivy. I bent down on one knee and extended my hand to feed the squirrel I expected to appear. A large brown county rat, not the long thin type, but the type with the humped back, reached out for my offering. I jumped back screaming. I realized County was not a place to approach on bended knee with outstretched hand.

The doors to Unit One opened into a long wide corridor, dark enough that it was never easy to see just how dirty or clean it might be. There was a noticeable change in the air the minute I crossed the threshold. Thicker, and heavy with the scent of people, that first breath of air always deflated my spirits a little. From this point forward, the journey to the cafeteria was an adventure. It was not an adventure students relished, especially for the sake of having a meal.

The corridor ended at one of the main thoroughfares of Unit One. One of the few things at County similar to other hospitals were the colored lines painted on the center of the floor. In other hospitals these lines guide people to various locations. Regardless of how the layout of County had evolved, these lines remained unchanged. Black, blue, yellow, red, green and orange - no one knew where any of the stripes led. Some things at County were older than God. These stripes were definitely in the running.

Another archaeological find at County were the ancient little men in volunteer aprons who ran the information centers. These information centers consisted of a battered card table and one folding chair. A dirty white cardboard placard bearing the word "Information" elevated this set-up to the equivalent of a hospital information center. I believe there were two of these "centers" in Unit One, but the one I saw daily was located near the door of the doctors' cafeteria. It was never clear whether the little man at the table was truly a volunteer, or a patient who had just wandered over and taken a seat. Some of County's patients have been in residence so long they may as well be volunteers.

Besides, I never actually saw anyone go to the information center for information. If someone wanted information, they would grab a harried-looking intern or nurse and ask for directions. Mostly the student nurses or interns would just visit for a moment or two with the man behind the information sign so he wouldn't feel neglected. Maybe that was his job, maybe he was supposed to receive information. I may have missed the point of the whole set up.

The stroll to the cafeteria usually contained two or three gomers. The word "gomer" is an anachronism for "Get out of my emergency room." The word was entrenched in the County vernacular on my arrival. I am not sure of its origin, but it was defined in a book that was being passed around by the interns and nurses, **The House of God**. County staff identified with the novel because it was set in a hospital almost identical to ours. It was also an inner city teaching facility and like County it served as the health care provider for the city's indigent and homeless. One thing was clear - gomers were a universal concept among hospitals serving the destitute.

My introduction to the term came at dinner time. A tall, lanky, red haired intern from Boston was entertaining the table with stories of his patients. "If I see one more gomer tonight I am going to scream. I believe it's true, they never die, like cockroaches, they will survive nuclear war." He took a long drag on his European cigarette preparing to elaborate on the horrors of his day.

He was diverted by requests to define gomer. "It's the guy sprawled on the floor that you had to step over to enter the dining room. If you are unsure, use your nose, they usually smell like urine. The old broads wear two or three dresses at a time and those ankle high stockings that cut off all the circulation to the feet. Their feet swell up like balloons." He was off on one of his favorite monologues.

Even the new students had already stepped over enough outstretched legs to know what he was talking about. Normally, a gomer is old, or at least appears to be old. Upon closer inspection, you may find a gomer who is only in their thirties or forties, which is particularly unnerving. But a gomer appears old, unhealthy, and has a ground-in dirt quality to their skin, much like the dark crevices of a trash bin. This is not dirt that comes off after one or two washings. This is dirt that comes from living in the streets or flop houses for an eternity.

Gomers usually have lice and if there are any open wounds, they probably have maggots. They smell of illness and decay. Their clothes are encrusted, and their whole being reeks of contamination. They are without resources. They are homeless. The constant presence of gomers was not only depressing, it was frightening. The fear comes from the feeling that only fate and good fortune separate you from the gomer. They threaten the most cherished of fantasies, that we are in control of our lives. For the exhausted doctor or nurse working in the emergency room, the sight of one more gomer crossing their threshold leaves them feeling drained. The nurses especially are the ones who will be called in to remove the clothes, the lice and the maggots in order to bring this being one step closer to humanity, so the doctor can bear touching him.

The thing about gomers is that they are not usually warm, friendly people, waiting eagerly for a kind word from a student nurse. More often they are angry, furtive, hostile people, more likely to growl than speak. Maintaining your emotional health while living and working at County requires becoming adept at not seeing gomers, unless they are your patient. I don't know how successful others were at this. It wasn't polite to ask, "Did you see that gomer?" Among close friends an exceptional gomer might raise a comment. Otherwise, I can only assume others saw what I saw, but each person was left to their own internal struggle with the view. Later, I would come to know gomers more intimately. At this point, the sight of a gomer put the unpalatable County food in perspective.

Many of County's patients are ambulatory, which means they are up and walking about. County patients are frequently tougher than patients in clean, nice, private hospitals. They are often sicker and they plan to survive, so they have to be tougher. Consequently, the patients that are up cruising the halls at County would be in intensive care at other hospitals. They may even be in intensive care at County, but they've still slipped out for a walk.

Patients with every type of bag or drain attached to them can be seen strolling the main corridors. Patients on heart monitors, I.V.'s and traction devices are all out for a little change of scenery. I have seen patients walking down the halls swinging their hemovac machine, which suctions blood and fluid out of wounds in the chest cavity, like a briefcase. These patients are all in hospital gowns, opened up the back, and usually bare-assed. Frequently, you can see from which orifice, whether natural or surgically induced, the tubes are coming. Being a patient in a large teaching hospital is one quick way to lose any sense of modesty. There just isn't time for such niceties.

I would pass into and through this parade of patients to enter the doctors' cafeteria. Surprisingly, the smell never varied much in the cafeteria, regardless of what they served. Years of overcooking vegetables and meat left a general aroma of mangled food in the air. County food can be summed up rapidly. It was dreadful. The food has been examined by the interns, cultured by the lab, and analyzed by the pathology department, but no one has been able to identify the origins of the mystery meat yet. As a matter of fact, no one had successfully discerned the ingredients in the topping on the pizza during the two years I ingested County food. As far as I know, no one has died from it. That's the best I can say.

Hospital life is a twenty-four hour a day, round-the-clock affair. The beginning of my day might be the exhausted close or the dragging middle of someone else's. At all hours of the day, newly graduated M.D.'s, now working at County as interns and residents, could be found fatigued and stuporous. They stared into their coffee with a dazed look on their face. In the beginning, this was alarming to me. I had been raised with the image of Ben Casey and Dr. Kildare. These disheartened, empty faces were not towers of strength or beauty. They more closely resembled children in need of mothers than heroes of modern medicine.

The alarming thing about these doctors was how frazzled and strained they looked. Doctors are not the cream of the crop. They are just samples from the continuum of the crop, like the rest of us. I was not surprised to meet the very bright doctors, and the occasional brilliant one. But I was totally unprepared for the mediocre-minded or even the dull-witted one. As a nervous student nurse it was very unsettling to find doctors who appeared to know little more than I did. Who would save the patients? I have come to learn that survivors are generally people who save themselves.

Some meals were quiet, isolated events, with only a few disheveled people sharing the cafeteria with me. Other meals were wild, raucous affairs. The lines were long, the tables were full, and spirits were high. These were fun meals, sometimes shocking or a little disgusting, but always interesting.

Dinner time was the most active. Evelyn, Susan, and I often ate together. Susan and I would get dressed, talking through our shared bathroom. Her appearance was unusual and intriguing. Though we were the same height and weight, her shape took a different form than mine. I am slender with muscles and curves; my bottom is particularly round. Susan's curves are in her breasts. She has nice moderate size breasts that droop in a pretty way. She has boyish hips and no ass. It gave her a completely different look than I have.

Susan's face is striking. Her left eyelid droops a little giving her a slightly cynical look. There is no mistaking the intelligence in her face. Susan looks like a woman who could devastate you with a word or two and she can. But she is not cruel, nasty, or bitchy. She is incisive and funny. I had many warm moments with Susan, yet I never really knew where I stood with her. She was not a person who naturally trusts others.

The most important thing on a busy night in the doctors' cafeteria is a good location. This could be a simple decision or it could be a complex sociopolitical issue. It depended on the circumstances of the moment and the variables involved. A friend would wave to us and gesture to the room available at their table. The simple could become immediately complicated if an undesirable person was also sitting at the table. An undesirable person might be a man that Susan, Evelyn or I were trying to avoid, or a woman that one of us couldn't stand, or just a garden variety asshole. These interpersonal conflicts were still relatively easy to solve. We would tell them we had promised to sit with another and then quickly find an alternative table.

It was the sociopolitical issues that got sticky. The population at County was as layered with strata as the caste system in India. Doctors were of course above nurses. Residents were above interns. The only people eating in the doctors' cafeteria were interns, residents, and student nurses. The rest of the hospital staff either didn't qualify to eat there, or had better options.

I fell under the broad heading of student nurse. By the end of two weeks, I had a pretty clear picture of the levels of strata within my category. First of all, there was the issue of male and female student nurses. Males are pretty well accepted within the population of student nurses. The men made up about fifteen percent of our class. As working peers, they are a wonderful addition to the nursing profession. Nursing is a tiring, demanding, difficult job; the women have mostly welcomed the men with open arms. Nursing, however, is not a highly esteemed profession. In the U.S., it is relegated to the level of "women's work." I guess this means it's a job too difficult for a man. The men I have met in nursing usually live up to its challenges admirably. Handling the pressures of the job is one thing; dealing with the stigma of being a man doing "women's work" is another. Some men, those with an incredibly strong sense of self, appeared to be unaware of the negative image. These men were like rare and special jewels. But most men experience the same types of internal doubts and fears that can plague me. These men would alternately sulk or rail about the blind stupidity of stereotypes. Their masculinity was threatened. Society branded them with the same adjectives it showers on the man who chooses to be a hair dresser, namely, that they are homosexuals, wimps, or incompetents. Perversely, they might even be labeled sex maniacs out to cop a feel. Some of the male nurses are homosexuals, but like society at large, the greater percent are straight.

I felt protective of our male cohorts. Most of my women friends felt this way. We had experienced enough sexism in our lives to know the pain of loosely flung labels. Any successful, competent woman who's been called a castrating bitch knows the no-win feeling of living outside of society's expectations. We thought of the male students as our men. They belonged to our group, and they were experiencing pain and confusion due to the cruelty of others. These men were variously our buddies, cohorts, companions, and lovers. The women tried to be loyal friends, sensitive to their feelings.

The problems arose in the hostility between the male doctors and the male student nurses. One sure sign that a doctor was a jerk was his expressing scorn at males who would do nursing willingly. A doctor might be bright enough not to denigrate nursing to a woman, but for a man to accept this form of labor was repugnant to him. A majority of males in our school retaliated by finding all doctors "egotistical assholes who didn't know shit." Female doctors were not unilaterally categorized. A woman was allowed the privilege of proving herself an asshole.

For the most part, females are attracted to males and vice versa. Egotistical asshole or not, a doctor is too juicy of a carrot for many females to ignore. Beyond that, there are also a large number of doctors who are truly fine people. Despite the feelings of many of our male counterparts, the population of male doctors was too large and enticing to be overlooked.

Many of the female nursing students were not great friends with the men in our class. So this dilemma of loyalty was not a concern to them. One of the classifications among the female nursing students was that of "doctor chaser". We who were not "doctor chasers" considered ourselves "women". The doctor chasers did tend to be the younger girls. They were mostly under twenty-two, and basically still boy crazy.

Some were out to catch a doctor and get married. Many just wanted to have fun with doctors, lots of doctors. In truth, they were a rather small percentage of the class. They were, however, a loud, colorful group, and drew a great deal of attention. This group was particularly irksome to some of the men in our class. These men came up with a few enduring phrases. One of the most caustic of these, J.O.D.M., was applied to the doctor chasers. J.O.D.M. officially stands for juvenile onset diabetes mellitus, a debilitating disease requiring daily injections of insulin. To the men in our group, J.O.D.M. meant juvenile onset doctor meat. It conveyed rather succinctly their opinion of doctor chasers.

A true J.O.D.M. is a wonder to behold. These girls would enter the cafeteria shining like a six karat cubic zirconium. Short skirts, tight jeans, infinitesimally short shorts, tiny T-shirts. Blue eye shadow, rosy pink cheeks, red lips. Hair that had been curled, sprayed, tossed, and fluffed. They can make eye contact and flash an engaging smile to as many as ten interns on a single pass through the cafeteria.

It took that much razzle dazzle because these interns were nearly dead. Thirty-six hour shifts had left them drained and just about worthless. But a determined J.O.D.M. could rise to the occasion. If she sat there and sparkled long enough, an exhausted intern or resident might soak up enough of her excess energy to notice how pretty she was.

From the very first day at County, I was amazed at the abundance of beauty in our class. A pretty face was the norm, a beautiful face was not all that rare. Our class held at least a dozen women I considered either striking or beautiful. A serious J.O.D.M. had plenty of competition from women who weren't even trying to look good.

All this doctor chasing affected my friends and myself very little. Sometimes it made for a pretty good dinner show. I only had a couple of dates with a medical student and one with a resident during my two years at County. I don't believe Evelyn or Susan ever dated a doctor. We weren't prejudiced against them. It just never came up. We spent our time mostly with the men in our class. Maybe doctors really do prefer J.O.D.M.'s. I do know those girls dated a lot.

I had not come to nursing school to catch a man, especially a doctor; of this I am certain. My mother had warned me early in life about the types of men to avoid. "Never marry a boy from a wealthy family or a doctor. The wealthy boy will be far too dependent on his parents, and doctors are boring, pompous, and keep terrible hours." There are exceptions to all rules and my mother would be the first to acknowledge this. But when it comes to judging people, she has an incredibly keen eye. Though after having seen the array of alternatives I have found to doctors and rich boys, my mother has probably at times regretted her announcement.

J.O.D.M. or not, I know very few females who relish being seen in public looking lousy. The trick in getting ready for dinner was not to overdo, a cross not borne lightly by Evelyn and me. Some women have a particular style of dressing and that's how they look. Sophisticate, ingenue, classic, vamp, I could never decide on a "look". I like them all. My weight stays consistent enough that I can wear the same clothes for years. My closet bulges with an eclectic collection of clothes. Evelyn's closet was as wild and unpredictable as mine.

We are spontaneous dressers. We dress for our mood of the moment. The frustrating part for me is expressing my mood within the confines of the situation. I have often wished that everyone would dress with a sense of humor. Clothes could be playful, wild, or subtle expressions of ourselves in the moment. Then I could dress as I like and still blend in with the crowd. Society does not seem eager to pick up on my concept of dressing. I loathe sticking out like a sore thumb. So I try to act out my whims as unobtrusively as possible. From the comments I have garnered over the years, I have not been too successful at blending in with the crowd.

Dressing for dinner, if I was in a hurry, was no problem. Jeans, a T-shirt or sweater, add some sneaks, and voila. It was when I had time, especially lots of time, that it got tricky. Time meant I could begin cruising my closet, exploring my mood. There is a moment when I pause, and ask myself what do I feel like wearing, that opens up a myriad of possibilities.

Cowboy is an enduring favorite for me. Punk and New Wave had just come in. I especially liked a twist of punk on a basic theme of cowboy. Silk or cashmere are also a nice counterpoint to boots and jeans. My taste in clothes, though odd, seems to be appreciated, sometimes for the strikingly good combinations I come up with, and sometimes for its comic relief.

The Old West didn't creep into Evelyn's closet at all. She frequently had an underlying tone of style and class, though she was likely to accompany a gray silk jacket with blazing purple toe nails. People didn't razz Evelyn as much as they did me. Her "don't fuck with me" look was that good. Still, we both suffered pangs at dressing for dinner. There was always the threat of being classified as a J.O.D.M. This worried Evelyn less, but she had that great look for keeping people in their place to protect her. At heart, I held on to that tiny fear, what if they are right? What if I am a budding J.O.D.M., and just don't know it? This nagging little self-doubt is what has kept me prisoner to other peoples' opinions to one degree or another.

Fully loaded trays in hand, we would stand, scanning the room. Some evenings there would be a "black" table. A group of black student nurses and doctors would all choose to sit together. This would cause a dilemma for Evelyn and to a lesser degree for Susan and myself. Evelyn was not an open person, baring her soul to the world. She would share privately with one or two people at a time. Some issues took us years to get around to. The issue of race was deep seated. It only came up rarely between us and always caught me by surprise. Probably that same lack of self-trust was at work silencing me on the subject of race with Evelyn. What if I was a bigot, and just not honest enough to admit it? So the wonderful exchange of information that could have taken place between us never did.

Evelyn's blackness meant very little to me. I saw it mostly in terms of aesthetics. Her skin is very dark and smooth. The feel of her skin was so soft, I loved to touch her. Evelyn's hair was like a brand new toy to me. She could do so much with it. Corn rows, braids with extensions and beads, Afro, natural, she always looked good. She tried to corn row my hair once and got nowhere. She said my hair had no body.

The physical package of Evelyn was so appealing to me, I gave no thought to the social aspects of living in her skin. I believe now that I was afraid of exploring our differences, for fear that it would separate us. I didn't want to jeopardize our friendship by talking about the differences between us. Evelyn may have felt the same, because we both avoided the subject a great deal.

It did come up occasionally. I sat in her room one day talking with her while she pressed her hair straight. She used a special iron I'd never seen before. The moment was familiar and comfortable to me, the things girlfriends do together. But Evelyn put down her iron and looked at me. She said, "I never thought I'd be pressing my hair in front of a white girl." She then came over and kissed me. I understood then that our love and friendship was harder for Evelyn than it was for me. I felt honored. I hadn't realized she was loving me in spite of my being white.

It has taken me years to begin to understand the nature of love. I grapple with it still. It is not enough for me to base my love of a friend or sexual partner on our shared similarities. I need to be able to share all my experiences with a loved one - to bravely explore our differences, as freely as we share our similarities. Unfortunately, during my years at County, I had not gained much clarity on my illusions of loving. I tiptoed around touchy issues with Evelyn. We spent our time exploring areas where we matched, not areas where we differed. So it took me years to understand that I am not a bigot, unbeknownst to myself. I am just another ill-informed white person, who at times says stupid things. Had I been brave enough to explore the topic with Evelyn, we might have loved each other and ourselves even more.

Evelyn had to choose where to sit. Susan and I knew she wanted to sit with us. We knew she liked us best. We three were best friends. Of course, none of this was ever spoken to. It was sort of a silent ballet, with Evelyn in the lead. Susan and I understood that Evelyn would be slighted by her black friends if she spent too much time with the white girls. Craziness, it was all craziness, but the fucked part is, it was also a reality.

Evelyn did have close friends among the black men and women. She must have felt very torn. She frequently expressed a strong sense of racial identity. Liberal whites can admire this, but they have no counterpart to it in their own life. Evelyn was stuck. A strong black woman, defiantly proud of her race, with two white chicks for best friends. She handled the situation fairly smoothly. About once a week, she would sit at the all-black table. Sometimes Susan and I, singularly or together, would join her there. The women at the table were always cordial to us, but I only felt truly welcomed by a few.

Eating with doctors, exhausted, overworked, dirty and drained, if they are bright, can be very entertaining. It's the kind of entertainment that's good in small doses. Like knock-knock or dead baby jokes, a little goes a long way. Although too much time spent with burned-out doctors can leave one callous, an hour for dinner is just about perfect. Sometimes they would bring props. X-rays were a dinner time favorite. Some doctor with a particularly bizarre set of x-rays would pass the films around. Everyone would take their turn holding the films up to the light. One could examine someone's ballooning aorta while chewing on mystery meat.

Marsha was a first year resident who specialized in gross diner time talk. She valued an attentive audience which was something I excelled at being. She always made room for me next to her at the table. Blond, short, chunky, and disheveled, she was the epitome of a burned-out doctor. Marsha was especially fond of dinner-time props. She usually carried specimens. Tubes of blood with purple or red tops were always jangling in her pockets. She was a particularly messy doctor and frequently spilled her work on herself. She also used her body as a message board, writing pertinent information about her patients on her left hand and arm.

Sitting next to Marsha and exploring her person provided a good fifteen minutes of dinner conversation. I had a hard time getting past the tubes of blood. We debated the issue often. I would point out the hazards of carrying around contaminated blood. Marsha would denounce any belief in the germ theory of disease. It would be two more years before any of us would hear about AIDS. Marsha's cavalier attitude seemed shocking, but not deadly.

Dinnertime did not consist of quiet, erudite discussions on medicine or philosophy. The hilarity almost bordered on hysteria at times. Sex was always a good life-sustaining topic. Marsha was particularly good at assessing men. We both had a broad range of tastes, with a variety of peculiar fancies. I later learned her tastes were somewhat broader than mine. She was even more astute at assessing women. A full cafeteria gave us plenty of material to work with. We were not pond scum. We managed to behave reasonably enough within ear shot of delicate male egos. But an arm's length away from any easily offended ear was all that was needed.

Marsha was gregarious. She knew everyone, and she wasn't afraid to probe for details. Not only could she assess men, she could give you the low down on them. People liked giving her the details, even knowing she wasn't very tight-lipped with the information she received. Dirty lab coat smeared with questionable stains, specimen bottles, and inky hands, Marsha was great dinnertime company.

It's time to leave the cafeteria for a while. If I don't, I never will.

Chapter Four

Mother Merlin Leads the Way

The curriculum at County was very structured; there were no elective classes. For the first year our class met three days a week for six hours of lecture in a large auditorium. In the beginning, we spent about two mornings a week working in the hospital. The time spent in the hospital increased throughout our training. Our last two semesters we were working three eight-hour shifts a week.

County has been training nurses for so long, that it has become a very efficient factory. This factory produces many of the best trained nurses in the United States. County did not employ progressive education techniques. The student did not determine the areas in which they would like to grow and expand. County taught you nursing, from the ground up. At the time I attended we were given a smattering of nursing theory to be contemporary. But this was not County's strong point. County's strength lies in teaching the realities of nursing. There is little candy coating. Nursing theory doesn't mean shit when you are suctioning six patients on respirators, and trying to maintain open airways in all of them.

A debate had arisen in nursing during my two years at County. Nurses wanted to be seen as professionals rather than as skilled technicians. I have never known more professional nurses than those coming out of County. Compared across the board to other graduating nurses, they are also the most skilled technicians I have seen. County is considered a diploma school. When you graduate, you have earned a diploma in nursing. There are only a handful of these schools left in the U.S. They are associated with large teaching hospitals. The current trend in nursing education was moving towards the universities, with students receiving a Bachelors of Nursing Science. The actual hands-on nursing took place at local hospitals. I do not want to enter the debate of diploma graduate vs. four year degree. The nursing profession is much more qualified to sort all this out. But, if I were in a tight spot caring for others, or needing care myself, I'd want a County nurse beside me.

Class was set up so that each semester you had a "Master Instructor" for the whole class. This instructor set the tone and delivered most of the lectures. We were also divided into small groups of ten for our clinical experience. I felt the universe had smiled on me in giving me Helen Merlin, R.N., as an instructor. A small black woman who had a look of knowing and accepting reality, Helen exuded love, intelligence, strength, and patience. Her sense of humor and well-grounded approach to life made her an absolute treasure. Every beginning nurse deserves Mrs. Merlin as their first instructor. I am forever thankful I was so lucky.

I had no fantasies about being the finest nurse to graduate County. Surviving, just graduating without killing anyone, was my main goal. County was a challenge I had come to conquer. Helen Merlin, R.N., was there to lead me. Mrs. Merlin never focused on me too much. She had more confidence in my abilities than I did. I felt like she never noticed my facade. When she looked at me, she saw a survivor and she left me to it. I missed the teasing concern that some of the others received. I assume I just didn't touch her heart in the same way.

Close to graduation, Sara, a member of that first group, and I, ran into Mrs. Merlin. She was concerned about Sara, worried that she would take on too much for herself. She gave Sara motherly advice and told her to take care. Mrs. Merlin then turned to me and said, "I never worry about you, you are going to do fine." It didn't feel like a compliment, just a statement of fact. I couldn't even feel flattered. I knew she was right. I didn't deserve her worry, I would be fine. But I missed her worry because sometimes concern feels like love.

I have at times tried to manufacture this concern for me from others, with little success. Upon hearing my fears of failure others reply, "You'll do fine. You'll pass the exam. If you flunk the exam, you'll still be fine." Even my mother, who loves me dearly, has a hard time working up concern over my anxieties. It frustrates me. My fears are as real to me as another's are to them. I want the same compassion for them. But healthy, well-adjusted people generally refuse to participate in fantasy, unless it is one of their own.

Nervous, but eager to begin, our clinical group met in a basement room, known as the lab. The room contained several hospital beds and mock hospital equipment. It was in the lab that Helen Merlin introduced us to the intricacies of nursing.

By our second meeting, we had begun calling her Mother Merlin. We followed her around, watching her every move. We trailed in her wake like a string of white ducklings. Noting how we grouped around her, hanging on each word, the Mother image was too strong to ignore. We were her chicks, confused and needy, fresh from the eggs.

We began with the simple things. Little successes, geared to build our confidence. It took two hours for us to successfully learn to read our thermometers. We picked up the pace though, as we went along. We had a fun group, playful, rowdy, and determined to learn.

I think I can remember our whole group. I know I've got at least eight correct. Gregory was the most prominent. His nursing whites were topped off by a full beard, a substantial Afro. and a devilish smile. He loved women. He was such a delight to flirt with no one even minded his attraction to every pretty face. We all happily waited our turn to snuggle up and hug Gregory. He would cozy up to me, drop a long arm around my shoulder, and breathe something wonderfully salacious into my ear.

Our group was a very physical bunch. Mother Merlin was tolerant of us constantly draping ourselves over one another. We were continually snuggling, hugging, tickling, and pinching. My friends told me other groups experienced much greater regimentation or competition. Mother Merlin nurtured us along, and we bound ourselves into a very close group.

Sharon was a real magnet for most of us. She was several years older than myself, my height, with a body that could stop a speeding truck. You didn't have to be a man to look at Sharon and know she would be a picnic in bed. Gregory just about lost his mind. Sharon had bright, sparkling blue eyes, a beautiful smile, and wonderful breasts. Wearing tight T-shirts, she would playfully jiggle her large round breasts at Gregory till he nearly melted onto the floor. It was almost cruel, the boy was so dissolved. Sharon had a heart of gold, but she was a little dingy. While she wasn't the quickest or the brightest in our group, she had outrageous behavior, and was funny, warm and honest - if you didn't like Sharon, you were probably dead. Certainly, she was the best thing to walk into many a patient's life at County.

Annie-Whammy, like Gregory, was one of the people Evelyn had introduced me to the first day of school. She was the youngest in our group, and all of us mothered her. She may have been nineteen like Gregory, but she wasn't going on thirty-five. She was immersed in all the confusion and complications that take place in one's life at nineteen. Ann was medium height, short blond hair, and undeniably chunky. She was also exceptionally funny, and not particularly pretty. Ann was alive, taking risks, blurting out her thoughts and feelings.

The name Annie-Whammy was not as cruel as it sounds. She was far too exuberant and lively to have a name as bland as Ann. She acquired the name very early at County. We had all gone out to eat and have drinks after school. This "all" included the fun people in my group; Evelyn, Susan, Gregory, John (another from our clinical group), and Cathleen, a friend of Ann's. It seems that after a drink or two, Ann caught the eye of a salesman at the bar. The man was somewhere in his mid-fifties and looked pretty dull-eyed.

The two of them began flirting. By the time he provided Ann with her second Margarita she was considering leaving with him.
This upset the men in our group terribly. After a few drinks, they were feeling overwhelmingly paternal towards Ann. They would flirt with her, hug her, and squeeze her, but they would never treat her badly. This salesman became Jack the Ripper in their eyes.

Gregory came up to me and persuaded me to talk to her. I was the voice of common sense, sound judgment, and all things boring. It is a part of myself I have tried to keep covert. The voice of reason never belongs to the person everybody wants to go play with. I have even been unkindly likened to Jiminy Cricket.

So I spoke to Ann. I spoke to the man. He didn't appear to be a rapist, only a dullard. She appeared to be determined. Short of my kidnapping her, the girl was over eighteen and free to go. In my best good advice voice, I told her to be careful.

Careful she wasn't, but safe she was. She took the salesman to her dorm room. Later that night we got the details. Ann had a brand new I.U.D. she was dying to try out. Mr. Salesman gave her a three minute test drive, exploded, and then petered out. Ann felt cheated. She yelled, "Hey, what about me?" Mr. Salesman had already given his all and it wasn't much. Ann told us her sad story with uncontrolled laughter. She immediately earned the title Annie-Whammy. Mr. Salesman was forever dubbed the Minute Man.

Not everyone in our group became fast friends. Serina was a person I never cared for. Something about her irritated me on sight. For no apparent reason, this woman drove me nuts. She was a very tiny, very pretty woman, with delicate Asian features. The first day we were to show up in uniform, Serina wore a red lace slip two inches longer than her dress. I instantly decided her judgment was shit, that she must be an idiot, and never forgave her. In truth, many people felt this way about Serina, and no one knew exactly why. Mrs. Merlin, tower of patience and tolerance, told Serina the slip had to go. It couldn't show and red was definitely out. But Serina was either unflappable or very dense. Next week's slip was black.

I have been known to be a little overly concerned about rules. Employers love me. At County I walked a narrow line, trying not to kill anyone in a world laden with danger. I conscientiously followed the rules just short of crippling my efficiency. Eventually I began to differentiate between the rules. I let go of the meaningless drivel that cluttered the process and held on to strong guidelines. But at no point could I forgive a red slip showing under a white uniform. Serina's flagrant disregard for rules and common sense damned her in my mind forever.

Serina managed to irritate nearly everyone but Mother Merlin. Serina didn't seem to care very much about the work or the rest of us. She never showed up by the side of a slower student to give a hand. She stood back from the rest of us, gave a minimum effort and appeared content. I always felt petty disliking her. My irritation with Serina was nebulous, constant, and unnoticed by her. Serina was just unaware, and it drove me nuts.

We had two earth mothers in our group, Maria and Sara. Both were warm, loving, gentle women, born to nurture. Maria's name fit her perfectly. With her round face, soft body, short curly black hair, and dark brown eyes, she was a warm mamacita with a laugh like crystal wind chimes. We were all lucky because Maria laughed freely. She had a relaxed natural attitude about life. Her situation at home with her husband and children was complicated. Things that would have caused me pain, confusion, and possibly embarrassment, she shared openly.

Maria's troubled family life was hung above her heart in the form of an ID tag. All County employees wear photograph ID tags. Maria arrived one day with her name tag severely mutilated. Her five year old son had taken a ballpoint pen and colored out his mother's face. Not content with defacing alone, he then jabbed the pen through her picture several times. Maria laughed and smiled a little sadly. "I think he's expressing his anger at me. We're talking about it every day and getting counseling." The badge, though painful, was funny. Her son had been so direct in his expression. You could see just how pissed he was at his mother. Maria wore that badge all semester.

Sara was a very quiet person. Our loud, rowdy group could almost obliterate her presence. Soft-spoken, no make-up, and long straight light brown hair, Sara had the look of an ex-hippie. All that was missing was the Indian bedspread skirt. Her home life was also complicated. Recently re-married, she and her husband were undergoing the tricky process of bringing their six children together as a blended family. Sara worked hard at home and at school. She had a gentle soul. This is why Mrs. Merlin worried about her.

John is the last person I'm absolutely sure was in our group. He was in his thirties, about 5'10", and skinny with lank blond hair. The hand he had been dealt for this life was not an easy one, and it never got any better. He had been a trucker and a laborer. His body held several tattoos. I believe he had served in Viet Nam. I can't remember if he was missing a tooth or if he just badly needed orthodontia. His eyes were small, blue, and a little beady. There is no kind and honest way to describe John's looks. He looked a little scary, unhealthy, and borderline psychotic.

John was one of those guys I just couldn't bear to have touching me. He was never politically astute enough to touch a woman without letting her know he was sexually getting off on it. It's a subtle thing; Gregory could drape himself all over me, while telling me delicious lies about how enticing I am. He was smooth with charm. It felt playful, affectionate, and safe. I think safe is the key here. John's touching didn't feel like affection, it felt like sex. It didn't feel safe, it felt sleazy. John was the kind of guy that would stand close behind me during a demonstration so he could feel my ass against his leg. And worse, he'd probably go home and think about it.

I reacted to John the way I reacted to many men that I was not interested in sexually, by playing the role of the prude. I would rather a man perceive me as boring in bed, than to have to face rejecting him. The part of me that is not a prude was offended at wearing this label. My strong sexual self resented being wrapped in sheep's clothing. It is not a simple thing, and I am not a simple person. The messages I sent out to men were as complex as military double speak.

Unlike John, the hand I was dealt for this life was loaded with good cards. Nothing about me is totally exceptional or outstanding. But almost all of my gifts are better than average, and the overall package of me is pretty strong.

"Life is not fair." My parents told me this very early. They repeated it often. At the time, I thought they meant, I won't always get what I want, or that I won't always have what someone else has. I could deal with unfair life on this level. As I grew older, I understood "Life is not fair", meant some children have alcoholic parents, live in poverty, are victims of racial discrimination, the list goes on and on. When I realized the tremendous discrepancy between the life I experienced and the lives of others, I felt very guilty. My interactions with John were a manifestation of all my mixed feelings racing around at top speed. Guilt is like a blender for me. When I feel guilt, my emotions and thoughts whir together. Logic and feelings all fly around, getting mangled into puree by the blades. The soup that remains is indiscernible mush. John pushed the high speed button on my blender.

Mrs. Merlin either didn't notice or wasn't concerned about our intra-group politics. Like obedient children we lived up to her expectations. We never treated each other badly, we were always kind and helpful. Mother Merlin brought out the good Girl Scout and Boy Scout in each of us. That is, each of us except Serina.

Chapter Five

Co-Ed Volleyball

The beginning of the third week of school a new sign caught my eye:

Night time Volleyball, 7:00 PM. Meet in the courtyard, Co-Ed.

The sign was posted on the wall of the dorm elevators. Our elevators functioned as an information network. Eager types placed signs here to tell you what was happening around school. Sarcastic types wrote caustic remarks on the signs.

Co-Ed. Twenty-six years old and still the word Co-Ed was charged with emotion for me. To play sports with boys! I had missed that opportunity due to teenage gawkiness. But now I could play a sport with men, volleyball. I was concerned. Suppose the men had no sense of humor about volleyball. Suppose they only wanted to win. My high school volleyball had not been too bad. As I recalled I was able to serve pretty well. But this was playing with girls, and our team definitely had a sense of humor.

I am not a natural athlete. My body looks more suited to a modeling runway than the tennis court or soccer field. But most of us want what we haven't got. I wanted muscle, strong arms and legs, agility, quickness. I wanted power and strength. I wanted to be a jock, a tom-boy, an athlete.

I didn't just want this a little. I wanted it a lot. Naked, I would stare into the mirror, studying the world's longest legs, thinnest arms, and a neck that is seventeen inches long. My mother and sisters consoled me. They told me the boys would eventually grow taller. They likened me to Audrey Hepburn. When everything looked bleak, some kind soul would remind me that Japanese men love long necks. Wonderful, I could be the tallest woman alive in Japan, where the men wouldn't even be tall enough to reach my neck, much less admire it.

I became exceptionally brave. I blocked out my fear of klutziness and showed up for evening co-ed volleyball. My bravery has its limits; I waited until the game was twenty minutes underway and then sidled over to the court pretending to have wandered by in my shorts.

Life does a wonderful thing when we aren't looking. We grow up. I hadn't grown up to become delightfully petite, or an incredible athlete. But I had grown up to be five feet eight, tall, but not gigantic, one hundred and ten pounds, slim, but not cachectic. The people on the volley ball court saw a relatively normal person and asked me to play. The side with fewer players actually greeted me eagerly.

Playing with men was as fun as I had hoped it would be. Toward the end of the game, they did get overly serious about winning and somewhat obnoxious. We would tease and harass these competitive males until they would lighten up, or sulk in silence. After all, it was summer. Evenings were hot, hormones were high, and we were here to have fun. Every excuse imaginable for fondling a teammate was used and abused. One man, Casey, had particularly active hands, and that first night wore a purple Bubble-Yum T-shirt.

He had shoulder length brown hair, a sturdy build, and stood about five feet, ten inches tall. This man was all over me. Hugging, squeezing, pinching, bumping butts, on and on. In my infinite worldly wisdom, I assumed this guy has got to be gay. No straight guy would cop a feel so openly. Gayness is something I have always been comfortable with in men or women. It was great to find a fun man I could play with. I bumped and rubbed against Bubble Yum all night. As far as I was concerned, volleyball was the greatest sport in town.

Neither Evelyn or Susan played volleyball much. It was my own private passion. I saw Bubble Yum around occasionally. He hung out with one of the girls in the class ahead of ours. Girl is an accurate word here. Her name was Trishy. Trishy was about six feet tall, big and boxy, with long curly strawberry hair. She giggled and squealed with the other girls. I had absolutely no use for Trishy. Her name alone canceled her out in my mind. She also served to reassure me of Bubble Yum's gayness. I couldn't envision Trishy engaged in anything but a platonic relationship.

I have never considered myself blind to the obvious. I egotistically consider myself astute. My people judgment is keen but odd; I usually hit the mark on the subtle things, but I may miss the obvious completely. Several days after my first volleyball game, I opened my door to find a note. The note asked if I was available for a date on Saturday and was wrapped around a piece of Bubble Yum gum. I was charmed. This required re-thinking the premise that Casey was gay, and finally giving him a call.

Casey needed a date for a close friend's wedding on Saturday. He promised a fun wedding with dancing and good food. I have been to a few fun weddings, a very few. Rarely can one count on a wedding being fun. I should have been wary when Casey asked if I was free on Saturday before telling me what he had in mind. I was too polite to renege once I had heard it was a date for a wedding where I knew no one.

Some dates are doomed from the beginning. The doom of our date went on for months. We had a long hot drive to the valley to attend this wedding. This gave Casey time to explain a few things for me. Actually, the person getting married was also a friend of Trishy's, a close friend. Actually, Casey and Trishy had been planning to attend this wedding together. Actually, Casey and Trishy had been going together for several years. They were having a sort of trial separation as of a week ago.

Casey was sure that I knew all of this already. He just wanted to be open and honest about everything. Murder occurred to me. I was on my way to the valley on the hottest day of the year. My nylons were sticking to my legs as I sat there pitting out my silk dress. I would soon be the surprise guest at a wedding where everyone was waiting to greet Casey and Trishy the Big.

From here on the day is as blurry in my mind as heat waves coming off a desert highway. The ride home was complicated by the fact that Casey was interesting and I liked him. He fed me more gruesome information about the girls in the dorm. Did I know Trishy and her friends lived on the seventh floor on the opposite end from me? He explained how angry they were at my "man-stealing" behavior. Interestingly, they weren't angry enough at Casey to stop talking to him. Casey was fun and charming. He came out smelling like a rose.

This was not a time in my life when I excelled at confronting people, especially men. More likely if anything smacked of romance, I became rather namby-pamby and docile. It was tough to resist the lure of pleasing a man who was attracted to me. Angry as I was at Casey, I did confront him. I told him he had manipulated me into a lousy position. I then sat down and listened to all his flattering explanations of how attracted he was to me. It had never occurred to him this might cause a problem for me.

I turned into putty in the hands of a man who could think; and would sell out completely to a man who told me I'm interesting. It never occurred to me that this could be a line. I assumed it came straight from the heart. It certainly went straight to my heart.

My heart acted like a railway switching station. Once it became involved the tracks of my thoughts were re-routed straight down to my gut, my storehouse for goodies like neediness, guilt, and insecurity. It can take anywhere from minutes to years for my brain to get back in contact with my thoughts.

I was lucky with Casey. He didn't touch me all that much. He was interesting and entertaining, but he had also spent three years with Trishy. This discounted him greatly for me. It's hard to get too worked up over appearing intriguing and complex, when one knows the baseline for comparison is Trishy.

I don't think Casey was all that worked up over me either. I believe he really loved Trishy. I think they may have gotten back together eventually. Casey may have just been hot for my bod - the last thing I would have expected, and probably the most obvious. We settled all of this fairly painlessly. I recall a total of three evenings spent together, and a few nice long kisses. We exchanged some warm moments, but no scars, and let it go at that.

Never before had I engendered the wrath of angry females. It is an amazing thing. Trishy had put on her armor and was out to mount my head on a pole. She was going to fight for her man. She gathered her army of giggling girls, and they formulated a plan. Trishy placed a late afternoon phone call to me. I was curled up naked in my quilt, napping like a cat. It was not a pleasure to be awakened.

My hello was soft and thick with sleep. Trishy's sharp voice cut through to my brain like a fire alarm. Peace immediately fled from my body. She felt we should talk. I should come to her room so we could confront the situation. Every fiber in my body was repelled at the idea of discussing this non-existent relationship with Trishy. I told her I wasn't dressed and wasn't coming to her room. But Trishy was hot and feeling strong. "Fine," she said, "I'll come to your room." I am extremely territorial. One does not invade my home, even if it is only a 12' x 15' cubicle. I told Trishy I didn't want to talk to her and I didn't want her in my room. Truer words I have never spoken.

I guess Trishy had felt the strong approach was best. Maybe, if she ordered me around, she would get my attention. She might intimidate me into behaving appropriately. I do not respond well to orders, unless I am being highly paid to do so. Having been told I didn't want her man, her presence in my room, or her voice on my phone left her no real grounds for battle. The confrontation was stymied. Trishy was S.O.L. and I was S.O.P., shit out of patience.

Bubble Yum Casey and Trishy rode off into the sunset, presumably to resume their tumultuous affair. I discovered I was left with a reputation. I was fast. I was ruthless. I would take a girl's man just for the practice. Pretty heady stuff for a woman who dated only two boys in high school. I had actually married the first boy I had sex with.

The idea of being perceived as a vamp was somewhat appealing. If I didn't have the psychic make-up to be free and easy, I could at least enjoy the temporary notoriety. My new image was flattering and exotic. I was surprised anyone would think me capable of "stealing a man." The image was short-lived. These giggling girls could only hold a thought for a month or so. I soon slipped back into the obscurity of my facade. I do feel the Bubble Yum affair left me tainted with a hint of intrigue at County. Occasionally I would attract someone's attention. An eyebrow would be raised. Their face would cloud, remembering they had heard something about me, but not quite remembering what.

I had a great time playing evening volleyball. I wasn't a star, but I did have a good serve. It wasn't a high over the head macho slug; I would have loved to have been able to do that. I hit my serve standing with my side to the net. I held the ball shoulder height and smashed it with my inner forearm. My serve was flat and fast. It cleared the net by a breath and went straight for their eyes. I wasn't very consistent. I frequently hit net balls, and I also had great streaks of luck. One evening I hit ten in a row, flat over the net. Our opponents instinctively ducked the ball flying at their faces. They whined for my removal from the court. My team yelled, "We're keeping her." I loved it.

Another man caught my eye during evening volleyball, and caught it much more tenaciously. Michael showed up for the games wearing baggy baby blue sweats. He was short, about 5 feet 4 inches, and looked like a child wearing Dr. Denton pajamas. I checked, there was no flap in the back. I wasn't too impressed with Michael until he sat on the ground, spread his legs apart and touched his forehead to the floor. It was pre-game stretching exercises and they got better once he took his shirt off. His body was compact, and firm, with a beautiful V-shaped chest. You don't get this type of build from exercise; it's genetic. It's a peasants' build for strength and endurance. I found it extremely attractive.

Michael's pretty chest and round ass were pleasant to salivate over during the games. In the upcoming weeks I would find out that Michael was bright, very bright. His mind and gut were a labyrinth of thought and feeling. I would eventually move toward Michael like a moth to a flame. Neither of us ever stood a chance.

That was weeks away yet. For the moment I was safe, basking in my unearned vampy reputation and enjoying the mindless bliss of co-ed volleyball.

Chapter Six

The Art of Nursing

Mother Merlin taught us many things in our first month or two of nursing school. We would go to the lab where she would reveal to us the mysteries of nursing. Then we would go into the hospital, where we would practice these mysteries on unsuspecting patients.

The Art of Applying A Condom Catheter According to Mother Merlin:

There are two types of catheters used on male patients. An in-dwelling catheter is a long thin tube that is inserted into the urethra of the penis. The tube runs up the penis and into the man's bladder. You know you're in the right spot when urine comes out. A small balloon near the internal end of the tube is blown up. This holds the catheter in place, and all is well. The process is a little more complicated than it sounds. It must all be done in a sterile manner so as not to give the patient an infection.

Condom catheters are a different story. Infection is not a problem here. Mrs. Merlin introduced us to condom catheters. We opened our mock sterile packets and explored their contents. I recall three main pieces: a large plastic bag for collecting urine, a long tube, and a rolled up condom.

Condoms are tricky things; for some, they are an emotional mine field. I do not believe it is possible to hand out condoms to a roomful of people without causing an uproar. Our group was no exception. We immediately regressed into hormone crazed adolescents. Condoms are great toys. They're slimy. You can unroll them, stretch them, taunt people with them. We were in idiot heaven for at least ten minutes. Unfortunately our condoms had valves on the tips for attaching the long tubes, so we couldn't blow them up. This was a big disappointment for John.

Mother Merlin was patient. She gave us time to collect ourselves enough so we could think. She explained the art of applying the condom catheter. To begin with, you connect the pieces together. This is easy and caused only a moderate amount of giggles. Next you clean the man's penis and apply the condom.

Theoretically, the condom is placed over the tip of the penis, then you unroll the sheath down the shaft - piece of cake. Penises are the strangest things. They have a mind of their own. I have found them to be either the most prominent or elusive things on earth. What is the plural of penis, peni? Nope,

I've looked it up in my American Heritage Illustrated Encyclopedic Dictionary. It's penises or penes, no pictures. Penes looks odd, so I'll stick with penises.

Anyway, a penis faced with a condom is a delicate situation. There are some men who can greet a condom fearlessly. These men usually discovered their sexuality before every female and her sister was on the pill. A really skilled technician can slip a condom on his cock without even missing a beat in the love making. You know you're with a pro when he opens the package with his teeth, keeping one hand free at all times for fondling.

Then there's the man who panics. His history with condoms is not good. Nature has forced him into a situation that is almost unbearable. Sex is no longer linked to her pregnancy in his mind. It is linked to his catching AIDS. I have seen this man weighing the possibilities in his mind. To die or to wear a condom. It's almost the same thing, for the condom is the death of his erection.

It's true, and it's sad. But my sympathy has its limits. I have used the pill, the diaphragm, the cervical cap, suppositories, and the sponge. I know birth control as if I had invented it. So do my friends. We are birth control smart, and we all hate it. I agree the condom has its limitations. It is also a welcome respite from my army of mechanical devices. Women have always known there is no perfect form of birth control. I am human enough to not mind sharing the discomfort along with the pleasure.

Mother Merlin's explanation was greeted with skeptical eyes. We all knew about penises and condoms. There's the dodger, the avoider, and worse, the shrinker. A penis with a true fear of condoms can shrink so small one needs tweezers.

Helen Merlin was smart. Her teaching was about real life, not theory. She told us not to worry about it. "If you keep messing around down there long enough, it will get bigger. Then you just roll the condom on." That made sense to me. I was always relaxed, friendly, and slow about my work when putting a condom catheter on a man. Mother Merlin was right. It's much easier that way.

Getting a condom catheter on is not the hardest part. Securing it in place without amputating a valued appendage is. Strangulation is the danger. Even without having a penis of my own, this sounds bad. One must secure the catheter by wrapping elastic tape around the base, close to the root of the penis. You must tape the condom, not the skin. The ends of the tape must be short of meeting by about one-sixteenth of an inch. This leaves room for expansion. The versatile penis that can grow large or shrink very very small is almost impossible to secure in a condom catheter.

Condom catheters secured, it was time to give our patient a shot.

Mother Merlin's Guide to Landmarks:

Contrary to popular opinion, giving an injection is much more involved than just jamming a needle into someone. Mrs. Merlin began by teaching us the landmarks. These are important when you are giving an injection that goes into the muscle. This is known as an I.M. injection, for intramuscular.

There are three main muscles one can aim for: the deltoid in the shoulder, the gluteus in the butt, and the quadriceps in the front of the thigh. Aim is important because all of these areas have other things located in them besides muscle. It's not good for the patient if you hit nerves or blood vessels. A careless nurse can cause serious injury to a patient with a poorly placed needle.

I took learning the landmarks very seriously. So seriously that my anxiety prevented me from being able to feel any bones in the hip. There is a triangular spot on the back of the hip, just above the curve of the buttocks. This is the spot you aim for. If all things are where they should be, you will avoid hitting the sciatic nerve.

Mrs. Merlin taught us the landmarks to find this safe zone, a spot where theoretically, I wouldn't cripple anyone. Though I might not be the finest nurse to graduate County, I really wanted to be a good one. I had fantasies of the type of nurse I wanted to be. I pictured myself giving a patient an injection so beautifully, that they would thank me. I wanted to give the most painless shot possible. I wanted to do nursing humanely. This was very important to me, something in which I could take pride. The more difficult a procedure was for a patient, the more skilled I wanted to be in performing it. I wanted my patients to feel they had been touched by a person who was present and aware: a person who would look at them and see them.

We paired up in the lab and began probing each other, as we searched for our landmarks. We started by finding the greater trochanter, a large protrusion on the femur, the long bone in the upper leg. We placed our hands on each other's hips, we pushed and felt around. We were all a little nervous. We were not very gentle. Fear rose in me. What if I were the only person in the world incapable of feeling the greater trochanter?

After some practice, feeling landmarks is not too tough. The bones are there. Obese people require more probing and occasionally some guesswork. I would hope their nerves were embedded as far below the fat as everything else was, giving me a little room for error. The fragile elderly man or woman with no meat on their bones made the problem more difficult. No one wants to hit bone when giving an injection. It's a creepy feeling. I was very careful and stayed shallow with these delicate frames. I never had the unpleasant sensation of feeling the needle bounce off the bone.

We were told giving a shot is like throwing a dart: the action is in the wrist. I don't know, since I've never seriously thrown darts. I listened carefully as Mother Merlin explained holding a syringe. Everything in nursing can be described in terms of at least fifty steps, all crucial. Omission of any step may lead to patient injury, death, or a lawsuit, but I will spare you the approximately forty-eight of the steps involved in giving an injection. In reality, conscientious student nurses learn and practice all fifty to one thousand steps in everything they do. Eventually all the little pieces come together in one smooth automatic process. At least this is what happens in nursing at its best.

My mental checklist for giving an injection was as lengthy as a pilot's take-off checklist. I went through the routine just as religiously. Determine the medication to be injected into the patient. Read all labels carefully, including patient's I.D. band. Know the indications and the contraindications for the medicine, know the side effects. Be aware of any negative synergistic effects with other medications the patient may be taking. Finally, know what a reaction to the medication will look like and what to do about it.

It's been years since I last held a syringe in my hands. The check list grows dim in my memory. Real life on the wards rarely permitted time for such lengthy mental gymnastics. But the feel of a syringe and giving a good injection remains. I enjoyed giving shots. I was good at it.

To get graceful injections, they must be practiced. The instructors gave all of their students equipment to practice with at home. Those concerned with following the rules conscientiously had their students work with unsterile equipment. Everyone was told to practice their injections on oranges. Mrs. Merlin gave the perfunctory practice on oranges speech, then handed us all sterile equipment. She even included vials of sterile normal saline, the basis of all fluid in the body. We had everything we needed. She told us to come back prepared to give our patients an injection. The unspoken was obvious; we went home equipped to attack our loved ones.

There was a shortage of loved ones in the dorm. This was early in our careers in nursing school. Friendships were new and tentative. Nobody was interested in being stuck by a practicing student nurse with sterile equipment. Michael appeared on the spot, the generous gentleman. He was a new friend. Michael was usually present at the evening volleyball games, and we had frequently been finding ourselves next to each other during lunch. He had come to my room once or twice for tea and cookies.

Michael was on stage whenever he was in my presence. He was excessively witty, charming, and entertaining. Finally I told him I was getting tired just watching him work so hard. All his breath came out in one big sigh. "It's only tiring you; it's killing me." With this announcement came some release. Michael's body quieted down, he became nearly calm. We talked about why; why was he dancing as fast as he could? Out came the world's most honest and painful response. "I wanted you to like me."

Meanwhile, I observed him, his hair, his eyes, his mouth. His hair was medium blond, curly, and too long on top. He fought to tame the curl. It wasn't too many weeks before I convinced him to trust me with his hair and a pair of scissors. With a new hair cut Michael looked like an ancient Greek statue, much like his namesake's David. He was four inches shorter than me. Michael was conservative and semi-religious. Our views on morality differed greatly. It was not a match made in heaven. It was made right here on earth, and probably on the hormonal level. Sensitive, emotional, bright, highly guarded, and beautiful to look at, he was more tempting than chocolate.

By the time Helen Merlin, R.N., sent me home armed with sterile needles in search of a willing arm, Michael and I were becoming good friends. We were still very platonic at this stage, not yet willing to jump completely into the abyss. Michael, Evelyn, Susan, and I were all gathered in my room. I was just dying to stick someone, and certainly unwilling to be stuck myself. My unwillingness to reciprocate greatly reduced the number of people willing to play with me and my new sterile equipment.

But Michael was a gentleman, willing to give without demanding reciprocation. Absolutely, it was usury. I did feel slightly guilty about it. But not so guilty as to deny myself the excitement of my first injection. I was smooth as silk. Nobody had to remind me of a step. I had it all down in my head. No nerves of anxiety at this point. I was sure I could do it well, and I stuck him.

It was a very tiny needle, which Michael appreciated. I did it pretty well. He didn't yell or wince. I think Michael and I had probably been salivating over each other enough by that time that he was willing to let me stick him just for the physical contact. Michael wasn't dumb. A first needle stick is a little like a first kiss. Donating his arm to me for such a cause secured Michael a place in my heart for life.

Mother Merlin's Aseptic Technique Test:

Aseptic technique is something nurses are taught thoroughly. This is a technique for working with a patient without transmitting any germs. Of course, the air itself in a hospital is full of yechy stuff so this is somewhat theoretical unless you are working in a sterile chamber. However, sterile technique properly done greatly reduces a patient's risk for infection. Surgery should be the epitome of sterile technique. It is also used for dressing changes, inserting indwelling catheters, delivering babies, and so forth. Aseptic technique is an art and nurses are probably its finest practitioners.

Maintaining a sterile field is a physical and mental puzzle. I enjoyed solving the riddle of how to make it all work. To begin with, you must have a place to set up your sterile field. Mother Merlin gave us a display of aseptic technique in top form. She brought out a large bulging parcel wrapped up in green cloth. She also had various small packages containing sterile gloves, 2" x 2"s, and 4" x 4"s. Two by two's and four by four's are small pieces of gauze doubled wrapped in sterile packets, and are used for a variety of purposes.

I delight in opening up packages of any kind. Looking at all of Mrs. Merlin's packages, I knew I was going to enjoy sterile technique. Here the game begins. The trick is to open up all these packages, arrange their contents in a useful manner, and even put on sterile gloves, without touching any of the contents with your bare hands, or with anything else that is not sterile.

Mrs. Merlin began with the big green bulging parcel. She placed the package on an over-bed table that she had rolled to the side of the bed. She removed the tape and carefully opened the folds of the cloth. Never touching the inside of the fabric, the sterile side, Mrs. Merlin quickly draped the table. Miraculously, the package's contents were now sitting on top of a table that was covered with a green sterile cloth. Everything had been kept pristine, untouched by germy hands. We now had a sterile field to work with. Mrs. Merlin moved on to the packages of gauze. She peeled back the top edges and flipped the gauze squares onto the sterile field, nifty. My excitement was building; I couldn't wait to play this game.

Carefully Mother Merlin slipped her hand under an edge of the green cloth. She created an impromptu sterile glove for her hand and arranged the objects on the table. There was a large basin and stacked inside it was a smaller kidney-shaped basin. The little basin held forceps and scissors. The basins were placed side by side, the other items were arranged for easy access.

She turned her side to the table but never her back keeping the sterile field in view. She opened a bottle of hydrogen peroxide and poured some into the kidney basin. Finally everything was ready and she opened the packet holding the sterile gloves.

Putting on sterile gloves without contaminating them takes a little practice. At that time, the gloves were double wrapped. A sealed envelope on the outside, much like a band-aid wrapper, protected the sterile paper inside that contained the gloves. A very nervous pair of hands can contaminate the gloves before successfully removing the outer envelope.

After her magical display, Mrs. Merlin explained the technicalities to us. She gave us plenty of packages to take home to practice opening. The following month we would be tested on our sterile technique. For the next few weeks, I practiced neatly flipping little gauze squares, and slipping my hands into sterile gloves without ever touching their outsides.

I was nervous about this exam. It was pass or fail, no curve, no mistakes. Either your field was sterile or it wasn't. Along with being taught sterile technique, we were also taught dressing changes. Dressing changes in theory are interesting to learn. Cleaning a wound in a sterile manner takes thought and dexterity. Over and over we practiced our technique on mock wounds. There was a constant and low level of anxiety for me in this. I knew that at some point we would be asked to do this on real wounds, ugly wounds, wounds I wasn't going to want to see. I was still holding out hope that it would be possible to avoid the gooey side of nursing.

However, we had to pass our exam on aseptic technique before we could go on to a more active role on the hospital wards. I showed up in uniform ready to take Mother Merlin's test. I was nervous but very confident. I felt not only would I pass, but she would probably tell me what an excellent job I had done. Whenever I have this strong solid feeling, I am about to land on my ass. It's inevitable.

We crowded into the corners of a small room while one at a time we were called to be tested. We watched, holding our breath, as our fellow students performed each delicate task. We silently moaned at each flaw in the performance. We wanted everyone to pass. I must admit watching Serina contaminate her entire field with one swoop of her hand was somewhat satisfying.

One woman, I think it was Sara, was doing a beautiful job. As far as I could see, her performance was flawless. Finally, she turned her back for just a moment on her sterile field. Fast and silent, Mrs. Merlin dropped a Kleenex on her field. Sara was intent. She went on with her task and never noticed the Kleenex. She failed, of course. It could have been a fly carrying hordes of germs. Mother Merlin taught us you never turn your back on a sterile field.

I perceived this exam as the first test of my nursing potential. Part of my lovely fantasy of clean nursing was my being able to slide through this test flawlessly. It's a "Catch-22" for me. If I am not experiencing performance panic, I may be engaging in a Disneyesque fantasy, with myself starring as Pollyanna. Mrs. Merlin held out the small box to me from which I was to draw out a piece of paper. This is how I would choose the sterile task I was to perform. With my Pollyanna spirit all aglow, I reached in and pulled out my task. I had drawn an inch round puncture wound in the anterior lower leg, not too tough.

The first part of the exam requires you to wash your hands. This has to be done in an approved manner. Your hands must not touch the basin during washing. You must wash several inches above your wrists. Dirty water from your wrists must not run down over your hands. So you must keep your hands elevated above your wrists, fingers pointed toward the sky, just like Ben Casey on T.V., walking around with his clean hands held up in an appealing to the heavens position. You must dry your hands on a paper towel. Throw the towel away, using your elbow to push the lid of the trash can if necessary. Then take another clean paper towel to cover the faucet handle as you turn off the water. We were working in a small conventional bathroom basin not designed for serious hand washing, so all this was not easy. Sinks in hospitals are deep and use foot pedals so the whole thing is much easier.

I bumped the inner basin once with my hand. My glow of confidence was dimmed, perfection was blown. I hoped that Mother Merlin wouldn't notice. It was a very small indiscretion. Mother Merlin might as well have been called Old Eagle Eye. She had a list of six septic indiscretions on my part. I failed the Aseptic Technique Test. She failed every single one of us.

In the following week, one by one, we all passed Mother Merlin's Aseptic Technique Test. It was our first big hurdle in nursing school, and eventually everyone drags their body over it. Mrs. Merlin taught me many things about the mysteries of nursing and about preserving dignity, my patient's and my own. She enlarged my sense of self-confidence while decreasing my cockiness. This in itself was a major feat. Mrs. Merlin called my attention to the little things, a fly on a sterile field may be an infection for a patient. I wasn't a new person, but I believe knowing Mother Merlin left me a better one.

Chapter Seven

Party Manners

About the end of the second month of school, the eager beaver types planned a party. It was to be a large social mixer of medical students, interns, and nursing students. People who are socially eager generally love theme parties. This was to be a luau. My friends all weighed the pros and cons of going to this party. A doctor-meeting bash with a luau theme does not rate very highly on the cool scale. If you play down the part about meeting doctors, and if you absolutely refuse to wear a costume, even a brightly colored shirt, it might squeak by with a three on a scale of one to ten.

Evelyn, and the more macho of our men, could not possibly sink so low as to attend a level three event, organized by go-get-'em nursing students. I was torn. I love the idea of parties. The thought of looking terrific, meeting fun people, and having a great time is very appealing. I always think of Cosmopolitan Magazine and their informative no-sense articles on parties, the likes of which I've never seen. Is the Cosmopolitan party a myth? Has anyone ever been to a party like that? I have been to perhaps two or three great parties. But these pale in comparison to a color photo of a "typical glittering holiday party" in ***Cosmopolitan Magazine***.

The fabulous Cosmo party may be a myth, if so it is a very effective myth - I have even occasionally bought a terrific outfit just in case a magical invitation should come my way. The fantasy party is losing its glow for me, like the prince on the white horse, I've waited too long for it to materialize. I will still give the occasional loving glance at those fabulous party dresses, dresses in which you couldn't possibly sit down, eat, dance or breathe. But I no longer look at their prices.

Clearly a nursing school luau ran no risk of transforming itself into the Cosmo fantasy party of my dreams. But every party is like a blind date; it is laden with potential. I was in luck. Susan was not above a party that ranked as low as a three on the cool scale. I admired Susan for having strong immunities to social pressure. Michael had no concept of a cool scale. He was in no danger of ever being mistaken for someone who was in the know of what's hot and what's not. Michael bought two tickets, one for himself, and one for Marcy, his closest friend since high school. At this time theirs was a platonic friendship, with strong, slightly possessive bonds.

Susan's sister Jennifer was spending the weekend with her. The three of us got dressed with our doors open to our adjoining bathroom so we could talk back and forth between the rooms. It was the summer of the strapless jersey tube dress. We all had one. I even considered wearing mine, until I got a look at

Jennifer in hers. Jennifer wasn't strikingly beautiful or exceptional, but she had all the components that make men drool. Certain bodies are the ultimate shape to fit a current fashion trend. Jennifer's body was meant to be wrapped in a clingy tube dress. One look at Jennifer, all boobs, tiny waist, and no ass, and I immediately returned to my closet.

Susan's eye was either not as acute as mine, or she had a stronger sense of ego. Susan wore her tube dress. So did about seventy other nursing students. I cruised my closet for the perfect summer party ensemble. Something definitely non-Hawaiian, something casual, yet sexy. It's a very delicate balance to look sexy without looking like you are trying to look sexy. God forbid people should see me trying to look sexy without succeeding.

I had a pale peach cotton skirt with delicate brown embroidery on it. The skirt fit snugly across my hips, then fell in soft gathers that accented my round bottom. The skirt buttoned up the front with the last button ending about three inches below my panties. The full skirt flipped open around my long tan legs. I wore a sleeveless brown cotton shirt on top. The effect was more subtle than a tube dress and I didn't have to worry about my top falling down.

I am a romantic cursed with bad party manners. My chit-chat repertoire is terribly limited. Cosmo has tried to help me with all their articles on "Catching that Special Man" but romance and blunt honesty are incredibly incompatible. I was also anxious about meeting Michael's friend Marcy. Though Michael and I had not crossed any sexual boundaries, I was starting to feel some heat rising between us. I wondered if Marcy would notice. I wondered if Michael had noticed. I wondered if I was mistaken.

The party had been going for an hour or so by the time I arrived. Everyone I knew that was coming was already there. Jennifer had not yet been completely gobbled up by the men. She and Susan were still available for talking. Michael had just arrived with Marcy. She was in a wheelchair, a result of an auto accident several years ago that left her partially paralyzed. My fears about getting along with Marcy were quickly put to rest. Our individual senses of humor blended well.

Relaxed and happy, feeling long-legged and pretty, I was beginning to enjoy this party. It wasn't quite the stuff of the Cosmo dream machine, but it wasn't too bad. The band cranked out Rod Stewart's "Hot Legs" with energy. Beside the dance floor was the blue glow of an Olympic size pool. The requisite tiki torches, piles of fruit, and spiked punch were in abundance. This was a fun party and people were up for it.

Michael, Marcy, Susan, and I began to peruse the food tables. Somewhere in the middle of the papayas, mangos, and passion fruits, Michael and I began to play with each other. It was subtle to begin with, innuendoes, salacious double talk, slow glances. Susan and Marcy were a little taken aback, but amused.

Susan had already decided I was overly focused on sex because of my intermittent mad dashes to my friend Jeff's apartment. I thought this was pretty normal. Susan found it a bit excessive. Evelyn and Susan had exchanged thoughts on periods of celibacy. Voluntary celibacy was something of which I had no concept. I had assumed ovarian death was the obvious repercussion to one month without sex. Statements to this effect labeled me in Susan's mind as something of a nympho.

She wasn't so shocked at my behavior as she was surprised to see it focused on Michael. He was not the type most women immediately think about bedding. He had no skills at flirting. He appeared overly serious. Michael's preference in literature was fantasy. He liked trolls, gnomes and knights in shining armor. He was the type of man who has read **The Lord of the Rings** several times, and actually wants to discuss it.

I have a keen eye. I watched Michael move. He was relaxed and comfortable with his body. It's important to watch the way a man handles his body. It's an indication of how he'll handle mine. I watched the way he ate. Michael was choosy and appreciative about what he put in his mouth. He took the time to savor his food. Besides the intellectualism and the overly busy mind, Michael was a sensualist - my favorite kind of man.

Possibly it was the two glasses of spiked Hawaiian Punch, maybe the stars were in the right alignment, but, whatever the reason, a "what the fuck" attitude settled right in and clouded my brain. This can be an infectious attitude. I began eyeing Michael like a rack of lamb and he caught the disease immediately.

We sat opposite each other in a group of about six people and proceeded to share a passion fruit. The ripe red fruit was oozing juice all over us. It was as close to foreplay as you can get in public without taking your clothes off. Michael slowly fed me one dripping bite after another. People groaned. Susan called us obscene, while Michael and I licked each other's fingers. Once the fruit was consumed, we dried our hands and went on with the evening as if nothing unusual had taken place. Our attitude mellowed. We became civilized again. My first brief taste of Michael was absolutely delicious.

I was now in the mood to dance. Michael was ready to focus his attention back on Marcy. The rest of the evening was a pleasant social swirl. While the band was on break, I sat alone and cooled my feet in the pool. In the movies this is the perfect set up. The heroine wanders off by herself for a moment of reflective solitude. Of course this is when she catches the eye of a wonderful man who dazzles her with his charm. In my scenario I insert Katherine Hepburn and Cary Grant into these roles as my prototypes. They are a hard duo to beat for style, wit, and charm.

In my real life experiences these are the moments I usually do spend alone, if I'm lucky. If I'm unlucky I catch the eye of an excessively pursuant Pee Wee Herman clone and spend the rest of the evening trying to shake him off. That was not my fate tonight. I was on some kind of a party roll. I felt elegant and lovely dangling my legs in the glowing blue pool. Right on cue, the cutest little medical student in the world sat down next to me.

Kevin was five years younger than myself, and truly adorable. He looked like a pre-teen movie idol. I later learned he was the heart-throb of the younger nursing students. When Kevin smiled he sparkled his dark eyes flashed and twinkled. His body was more Kevin Costner than Arnold Schwarzenegger. Kevin's chatter was socially adept and very pleasant. By now he's probably a budding politician or a successful gynecologist; either would suit him beautifully.

I spent the next two hours dancing with darling Kevin. I can see how men lose it for very pretty women. It is a rush to see this incredibly beautiful face beaming at you. There is even a vague sense of "I can't believe this is happening." The novelty of a movie star face is nice. It's like an ice-cream bon-bon covered with chocolate - a great snack, but not life sustaining. When I'm hungry for male companionship, I don't want a bon-bon, I want a meal. On this night, I was definitely hungry. I went to sleep with dreams of Michael licking my fingers.

Chapter Eight

Angel in White

Once we passed Mother Merlin's aseptic technique test, we were given the privilege of performing more complicated tasks on the wards. A few in our clinical group, mostly the men, found this very exciting. Now we would finally get down to real nursing. I was not so energized by this prospect.

Our clinical group met on the wards at seven A.M. on Monday, Wednesday and Friday. I would get up at five-thirty to shower and dress. Putting on my uniform was the first non-self-enhancing act of the day. One woman out of a hundred looked good in this uniform. Good is even too positive a word, one woman out of a hundred looked not too dreadful in this uniform.

It was a sad, sack-like affair of stiff white cotton polyester that would ball up in a very unappealing way. I was never able to determine a bust size that looked well in this dress. Bust sizes 35" or under left the bodice concaving on your chest, deflating one's ego in a horrifying manner. Bust lines of 35 1/8" or larger caused the dress to bulge and pull at the buttons, adding at least ten pounds to the wearer's appearance. Slender women looked like shapeless sticks, average women looked like pudges, plump women looked like whales. This dress was a self-effacing wonder of modern technology. Any ego that remained after putting on our uniform was finished off by slipping your feet into a pair of orthopedic nursing shoes.

I found a shattered ego could be avoided by turning off the light before looking in the mirror. I practiced this system religiously and found myself much more comfortable in my uniform. I usually shared a rushed breakfast with Evelyn before meeting my group on the unit. We would meet in the break room which was a cubbyhole with a few chairs. Mother Merlin would assign us our patients and tasks. At this point we were assigned only one patient to work with a day. Later we would work our way up to caring for four to six, depending on the severity of patients' condition.

First semester all students worked on general medical or surgical wards. Patients on these floors at County were frequently sick enough to be in critical care or step-down units in private hospitals. Once we had been taught the basics of performing complicated tasks, Mother Merlin threw us right into the pool to sink or swim.

Mrs. Merlin arrived on the ward early, carefully selecting and assigning our victims. Patients were chosen by the challenges they would present us. I was the first in our group to sample the pleasures of inserting a Naso-gastric tube. An N.G. tube derives its name from its origin and destination. The tube is run up the nose, down the esophagus, and into the stomach.

Mrs. Merlin had found me a tiny, bird-like little woman named Anna. Anna was seventy-two years old, disoriented, and emaciated. Because of her disorientation she had to be tied to her bed with soft restraints. She was confused, agitated, and assaultive. The only way to ensure Anna getting enough nourishment was to force feed her through a tube in her nose. This did not bring Anna any joy.

My patient had been discovered by her landlord in a flop house on skid row. She was unconscious, starving, and losing a battle with basal cell carcinoma. The carcinoma had eaten away Anna's nose and part of her upper lip. What remained was blackened, and in the process of further decay. My first thought on seeing Anna was why? Why are we doing this to her? Where is the dignity and humanity in this process? The only point left in Anna's existence appeared to be to give me experience in inserting an N.G. tube. We weren't easing and making gentle her exit from this planet. We were going to fight her every step of the way.

These are touchy issues, the quality versus quantity of life. At what point are we intruding and forcing our helping hands unwantedly on another? Do we have the right to invade Anna's privacy, to tie her down and insert our tubes, to prolong a life of pain? Certainly Anna did not give us her permission. She fought, and struggled, and struck out at us, every chance she could. These were taken as signs of her confusion. I was not convinced that these were not signs of her clarity of thought, expressions of anger to which I felt she had every right.

This procedure was painful for me on many levels. Physically, and emotionally, approaching a half-eaten face to insert a tube into a hole of devastation took great courage and control on my part. Anna writhed in her restraints. I was determined to treat her with as much integrity and respect as possible. I controlled my voice, I looked her in the eyes, I talked to her.

My first words were an apology. "Anna, I'm so sorry. I know you don't want this." I explained what I was going to do and what she could do to make it as easy as possible on herself. Her eyes were wild. I don't know if she understood anything I said.

I completed my task as quickly and competently as I could. Sharon and I then gently gave Anna a bed bath and changed her sheets. The procedure was reversed the next day. It was Sharon's turn to acquire the experience of inserting an N.G. tube.

The stories of treating indigent patients are endless and spiritually exhausting. The callousness developed by many professionals is a defense system to keep their psyches intact. Not all indigent patients are dying. Many are alive and are going to keep on living. Being part of the machinery that disempowers and dehumanizes these people was an extremely conflicting experience. I wanted to learn to put in an N.G. tube. The price of further traumatizing Anna felt like an awfully high price to pay.

Others say, we are the Saving Angels, doctors and nurses, fighting disease and pain. It is our duty to heal the sick, whether they want it or not. I can not live with this philosophy. I would pray, "Dear God, please don't let me wind up indigent and ill in a county hospital. Don't leave me in the hands of well-meaning doctors and nurses devoted to intervening in my natural life processes. Please, let me die in peace."

Chapter Nine

This Is Just A Friendship,
And Other Sweet Lies I Have Told Myself

Three-quarters of the way through first term we were given a two week break. It was the end of September. I don't remember why we were so lucky as to get this break; we weren't given many. County ran its nursing program on a year-round basis, no summers off, no long breaks.

A week or so before vacation, people began making plans. We had been together long enough to lay the groundwork for a social network, but not yet long enough to develop much emotional intimacy. Michael had decided to go backpacking in the high Sierras for eight days. He was going with a group of people and invited me along. I probed for details: Were these close friends, did he like all the people going, how many in the group? Probing for details struck Michael as slightly rude on my part. What did it matter? It was a group of people and I was being invited to join.

It matters a lot to a person with congenitally bad party manners. Eight days in the mountains with a random group of people could easily degenerate into prolonged party hell. The details were not encouraging. "You know, a group, six, eight, ten, whoever wants to come along." Michael explained one of the beauties of backpacking was to have a communal atmosphere, open to anyone who wanted to join.

I own up to it, I'm a snob. If a snob means you are picky about the people with whom you associate, then I'm a class one snob. People tend to sense this about me and many don't appreciate it. I have few friends, but they each bring something I value to my life. My friends are usually people on the periphery of the mainstream. Or as my mother might delicately put it, "kooks" and "off-beat types."

Appealing as backpacking with Michael was, there was no way I was going to put on a pack and walk into the woods for eight days with a random group of people. I exposed myself to Michael as a snob and confessed my picky nature. I told him the only person I had the least bit of interest in backpacking with was him.

This had two effects on Michael: from a sociopolitical perspective he disapproved of me. What about universal caring toward all mankind? What about treating everyone as equals? What about unconditional acceptance of others? I confessed I thought all that was shit, and people should be judged on their merit.

Michael and I both had a hidden agenda. This wasn't just a friendship. Philosophies aside, we wanted to be together. This is the time in a relationship when it serves one well to listen very carefully. In the span of fifteen minutes Michael and I had exchanged a wealth of information about our views on life. It was rather vital information on very discordant views. Hormones are powerful things. They can be a blinding, driving force. Michael and I were in high gear hormonal overdrive. Our eyes and ears closed down into tiny little apertures. What ever information did sneak in our brains quickly shuffled around into something more palatable.

It's magic, it's romance, it's chemistry. It's all done right before our very eyes. An emotional sleight of hand, now you hear it, now you don't. In the amount of time it takes me to inhale the scent of him, I can rearrange every word out of a man's mouth.

I am able to see my women friends more clearly because I don't have a hormonal surge to blind me. Other factors come into play to cause me to tune out vital pieces of information, like neediness, seeking approval, and slimy little things like that. But none of these have the powerful blinding capacity of a good hormonal surge. Therefore, I end up with a higher level of compatibility with my female friends, and friendships of greater quality, and longer duration.

Through all of this I have had the lack of insight to wonder what is wrong with men. How is it I know them so well in the beginning, only to have them turn into strangers I don't even like? The men have every right to be pissed as shit. So do I. But we ought to be pissed at ourselves, not at each other. For me, most often the deception is an internal process, not an external one.

The second effect my announcement had on Michael was flattery. This was not my intention in revealing my snobbery. Once he finished spewing out platitudes, Michael began to glow. My words had sifted down past his brain and reached his heart. His heart forgave me for being politically incorrect. His mind got mired down in the warm gooey softness of his feelings. He had heard correctly; Michael was the only person with whom I had the least bit of interest in going backpacking.

Flattery is as contagious as any other social disease. Michael's glow spread to me. I was flattered that he was flattered. Warm gooey softness now enveloped us both. Our minds had lost the battle. Now was not the time for a philosophical dialogue. We smiled and sparkled. We made plans for a backpacking trip for just the two of us.

Chapter Ten

This Is Just A Friendship, But I Think I'll Pack Some Birth Control

One good thing about birth control is that it makes us examine our intentions. The more immediate a form of birth control you use, the more closely you have to examine your intentions. A woman using an I.U.D. can go a year or two before examining her intentions to have sex. The Pill, like the I.U.D., gives a woman the luxury of engaging in sex without prior thought of the act.

If you use a form of birth control that is more immediate, then you have to take more responsibility for your behavior. This is what they call taking out all the spontaneity, or killing the romance. And they are right. It is undeniable premeditation to pack your birth control for a trip with a friend. There is something defiant, practical, and resolute in tossing your diaphragm into your purse. You know when you place that diaphragm in your purse there is no way you can feign surprise when you pull it out. At least not and maintain any sense of personal integrity.

I had to be realistic about this. Though we had not even shared an intimate kiss, the chances of our having sex on this trip were at least fifty-fifty. Except for the slimy types that drool and stare, I have a hard time guessing when a man is sexually attracted to me. I flash back on days in junior high school when nobody wanted to neck with me, and assume things have remained the same.

I had mixed feelings as I searched through my sperm control arsenal. Michael may have no desire to have sex with me. My sexual advances could be seen as a gross infringement on our friendship. No problem, I won't make the first move. I'll be passive, sweet, and platonic until he indicates his interest. Then cool as can be, I'll whip out my birth control device. Somehow the romantic glow fades at this point in the fantasy.

Loss of romantic glow is preferable to the loss of a potential eight days of fun sex in the mountains. It is also preferable to pregnancy. I felt sadness at the unavoidable loss of spontaneity, romance, and innocence. I distracted myself with concerns over which form of birth control is most suited to backpacking.

There are various issues to be considered. First of all, there is a finite amount of space in a back pack so you have to think small. Secondly, there are no bathrooms with hot showers, so you have to be prepared to rinse out your diaphragm in the river, or worse, a tin cup. Thirdly, there is the issue of ecology. Backpackers have intense feelings about screwing up the ecology. What you pack in, you must pack out. This limits the appeal of condoms.

I settled on Semicid suppositories as the perfect birth control for backpackers. That is if you are comfortable with a less than ninety percent reliability. I figured I'd go with it. The gods couldn't be that cruel. Semicid are small, slender, bullet-shaped suppositories packed in a neat tiny container that holds twelve. A week of backpacking bliss in a two by three inch container.

The less important details I left to Michael. He plotted our route and assessed our food needs. My input on the supplies list was to request one chocolate bar per day, and a cup of hot chocolate for mornings and evenings. Michael was very practical. We each carried eight zip-lock baggies. Our baggies contained granola, dried fruit, nuts, and a chocolate bar. This was lunch. Seemed a bit meager to me. The rest of our food was stuff like Top Ramen and Kraft Macaroni and Cheese. This was clearly not the gourmet tour.

The night before departure we prepared our packs. I had never backpacked before. I borrowed my pack from a friend in the dorm. It was exciting to drag out all our stuff and begin cramming it into our packs. Michael was not a sexist. We would share the weight as evenly as possible. I was no wimp. At least my facade was no wimp. Anything Michael could handle, I could handle. "Pack it on me," I said.

"Pack it on me" was the last unburdened thing I said for eight days. The laws of physics cannot be avoided. Biomechanically I am not well designed for hauling heavy weights long distances up mountains. At this point in time I had not yet discovered the wonders of Nautilus machines and the joys of strong arms. My bones are long and slender. My five-eight frame weighed a hundred and ten pounds. My pack weighed almost fifty pounds. A well-fitting pack distributes the weight mostly on your hips. An ill-fitting borrowed pack leaves the weight precariously teetering on top of your shoulders, behind your head and neck.

Michael's short sturdy one hundred and sixty pound body was built for backpacking. He looked great carrying a backpack, solid and strong. I felt like a gazelle balancing an elephant on my head. If I leaned an inch too far in any direction, my feet broke into a run trying to stay under my pack.

I crossed the lobby of the dorm following behind Michael. I wanted to look like my friends that I admire, when they backpack. I wanted to look solid, aglow with health and strength. I tried to look casual and relaxed as I made my way across the lobby. I kept my feet wide apart for balance. I tried not to waddle. Clearly, if I wanted to get laid this trip, I would have to keep Michael in front of me at all times. The less he saw how I looked with a pack on my back, the better.

After a treacherous fifteen minutes, we reached Michael's car. He had one of those little bitty Hondas that look like a shoe box with wheels. It suited him perfectly. With a strong heaving swing of his body, Michael shifted his pack off his back and into the rear of his car. I observed this. I stood erect, and smiled casually. I pretended not to notice the sweat running down the back of my neck and between my breasts. Michael offered me a hand, removing my pack. "God, I'm saved," I thought. I calmly said thanks and turned my back to him while unbuckling the hip belt. My jaw dropped in relief as I felt Michael lift that gorilla off my back.

Only a six hour drive and we would be at the base camp in the High Sierras. I still felt I could do this. I will get past the pain. I will learn to balance that monster without toppling forward. I will learn to do this or I may die in the mountains. I didn't admit a thing to Michael. Everything was just fine. I couldn't wait to hit the trail. I was that most venerable of creatures, a mountain woman.

We arrived at the base camp around six o'clock and set up camp. I had all the right outdoorsy, nature person stuff. I had a nicely worn North Face down vest, well broken in Raichle hiking boots, even biodegradable soap. What I didn't have was a stove, a tent, a knife, or any idea of how to take care of myself in the woods. I was totally dependent on Michael and his skills.

Setting up camp was not complicated because we weren't going to use a tent. Hopefully we would never have to use a tent if the weather stayed nice. Michael said this was our hope because our tent was a two man tube tent. The disdain in his voice made it clear to me that a tube tent is not a good thing. I had no idea of what was wrong with a tube tent, but I understood we were to hope for mild weather.

At eight o'clock the next morning we hit the trail. The first part of the trail was designed to accommodate the lowly day hiker. The day hiker is not a free spirit taking off with only the essentials, out to commune with nature for a week. The day hikers frequently consist of families, radios, teenagers, and coolers. Coolers holding as much beer as two men can possibly haul in two to four hours. The distance day hikers trek is inversely related to the amount of beer they pack. This is of course a jaundiced perspective. It is the perspective passed on from the experienced backpacker to the novice. I was eager to gobble up any information that would help me appear to be a seasoned backpacker.

Sneering at day hikers helped keep me focused off the pain. Vice-like shoulder pain was the dominant sensation I was experiencing. An inescapable weight bore down on my shoulders and upper back. A metal bar dug into my lower back. It is amazing to think I had voluntarily strapped this contraption onto my back. I have the ability to be very stoic when the only alternative is constant whining. I strongly believe people that whine should be shot and put out of their misery. So I was quiet. I trudged along behind Michael, head down and sweating. I saw a great deal of the path.

We did take breaks. I felt light and free as if released from prison. Short breaks I would lean my back against a tree, letting the tree support my pack. The cool breeze would dry the sweat on my chest. I could lift up my head and look around me. The view, the smells, the sounds of the woods, all nurtured my spirit and brought me joy. I loved being in the forest. I felt peaceful and exhilarated at the same time.

Lunchtime was great. We took off our packs and our boots. We sat by a stream and hung our feet in the cold water. Michael was a good packing partner. He didn't run his mouth the whole time. We stayed quiet and each enjoyed the view by ourselves. Exertion is the perfect aperitif. Cheeze Whiz would have been as welcomed as aged Brie after four hours under my pack. A chocolate bar under these conditions was almost a religious experience.

It was actually worth the pain, and there was a considerable amount of pain. Setting up camp, washing in the stream, building a fire was worth it. We saw very few people after lunch. There was no one within sight of our camp. I was absolutely exhausted by the end of our first day. I was also totally happy to be where I was.

Michael and I heated up something gooey and disgusting to eat. It tasted great. He then began the project of hanging our food. Hanging your food is what you do when you camp in areas with bears. We had read signs warning people to take precautions with their food. The trees also had claw marks on them, probably from the bears trying to get to the food hanging on the branches.

Michael took this as a personal competition between himself and the bears. There were rules to the game. You had to hang everything that smelled even remotely like food. This included chapstick and toothpaste, two things I like to have around at night. You had to hang your food while you still had enough light to see what you're doing. You had to keep in mind Mama bears and baby bears. Mama bears can reach higher, baby bears can crawl out on smaller limbs. Michael was sure Mama bears taught baby bears to do this.

This challenge would absorb Michael for a good hour every night. It was serious work. Losing your food is bad when you are one day out, it's terrible if you have already hiked four days into the mountains. Michael got very creative about it. He worked out pulleys and lines. He suspended our food in the most unusual ways possible. If he had died in his sleep, I probably would have starved to death.

This food hanging business gave me time to relax pack-free and watch Michael in action. Overcomplicating procedures is a strong indication that a person possesses a busy mind. My guess was Michael had a ruckus going on inside his head. He examined every tree in a fifty foot radius of our camp. He assessed the height and strength of their branches. I watched his legs because he was wearing shorts. Tight shorts, so I also watched his ass.

My thoughts as I watched the muscles in Michael's ass tense and relax, were more appreciative than sexual. Once I removed my pack and pulled off my boots, I became immobile. My body felt like it had just been released from six hours on a torture rack. I had collapsed next to my pack. Michael gave thought to where we should roll out our sleeping bags. I nodded attentively as he searched the terrain. He moved rocks and evaluated the degree of slope, while I reached over, untied my bag, and kicked it open beside me. Michael decided the correct slope and base for his bag could be found next to mine.

I was not able to remain immobile. Eventually I had to get up and find a private place to pee. Feet that have been recently released from boots are loath to put on shoes again for at least twelve hours. I was a cripple. My shoulders were so painful, I couldn't believe they weren't bleeding. My low back felt like someone had ben beating me with a hammer. Even the motionless sex of the missionary position might have killed me. I found a private place in the woods. Then I returned to camp praying I would not have to move again for eight hours.

Lying in my bag staring at the stars was magical. I felt no pain as long as I remained motionless. Michael and I talked until our voices faded, and we fell asleep.

Crawling out of a sleeping bag on a cold wet morning is treacherous work. I dragged my cold damp clothes into my mummy bag. I spent fifteen minutes trying to maneuver my long gangly limbs into my clothes, without exposing any skin to the cold morning air. My approach was the weenie method; Michael's was manly. In a macho, self-sacrificing manner, he jumped into the cold morning air and his freezing clothes.

After a quick breakfast, we repacked our stuff and were on the trail. Today was my day to become intimate with switchbacks. Switchbacks are a form of sadistic hell, created to torture novice backpackers. I faced a never-ending trail of tight zig-zags climbing up the stone face of a mountain. There were no trees to shade the sun beating down on my head and shoulders. The glare from the rocks assaulted my face and chest. Sweat ran off my brow, down my nose, and into to my boots.

Our trek seemed endless. We spent at least three hours performing as beasts of burden for the pure pleasure of it. My view was limited. Stooped, with my load and my pain, I saw little. Grey granite sparkling with blinding patterns of sunlight and Michael's tan legs encompassed my entire field of vision. Observing the shortening and lengthening of the muscles in Michael's legs and ass was my only form of diversion from the pain.

I studied my view. The rhythm was hypnotic, a forward reaching with the right leg, muscles tensing, bulging in the calf ready to accept his weight. The left leg reciprocated with a lengthening and relaxing of the muscles. Tense, release, tense, release, the rhythm massaged my brain. Massaged my brain right off my pain and into fantasies of sex.

I grew very partial to these legs and this ass, the beauty of their power and movement. Sexual fantasies are about the best escape I know of. I can avoid almost any kind of pain or tedium, except hunger, with a good sexual fantasy. I felt a little guilty mentally abusing my friend in this manner, but not guilty enough to cease and desist my imaginary ravaging of his body.

The rest of our second day on the trail is a blur, lost somewhere in fantasyland. My next clear memory is lying in my sleeping bag next to Michael staring up at the sky. It was a beautiful night, there were shooting stars. I still had no clue to whether or not Michael was romantically interested in me. I could see three options: he might be shy, he might not be interested, or he might be waiting for the perfect moment. I spent the time worrying, "Is this man ever going to kiss me?"

Yes. Michael rolled to his side, leaned over me and kissed me. That was all that was needed, our bodies took over from there. Many people believe the first exploratory sexual encounter with a new partner is the most exciting. The thrill of a new conquest has been highly touted. This has not been my experience. The first time can range from so-so to blissful, but I have found it always improves from there. As our kissing under the stars became more passionate, I dragged myself from his arms and over to my backpack. Naked in the moonlight, I searched for my birth control. "Where did I pack the damn stuff?" Panic ceased, my brain cleared, and I remembered to check the front lower pocket of my pack.

Michael was an anti-abortionist, one of our many disparate views, so he had made an effort to be thoroughly versed on birth control. I returned to our bed, Semicid in hand. Michael saw my package and announced in an intellectual, well-informed tone, "I believe we have fifteen minutes to kill." It was true, Semicid do not become effective until fifteen minutes after insertion. I responded that I didn't equate foreplay to killing time. Michael saw my point and happily proceeded to kill fifteen minutes with me.

The flavor of our trip didn't change drastically. We just became warmer, sweeter, and more relaxed. We had now completed the pact between us. We would no longer focus on subjects that were divisive. We would focus on all the ways that we agreed and how we were connected to each other. And so began a joyful, loving, thoughtful relationship

The duration of our pack trip was eventful. We hit rain, hail, and snow. I learned first hand why one hoped for good weather when packing a two-man tube tent. In the pouring rain and wind, we slept in a contraption the equivalent of a large Hefty bag. It was the size of two lawn and leaf bags laid end to end, with both ends open. When you breath in this type of a set-up, the condensation that forms drips right back down on you. We slept cold and wet in soggy sleeping bags.

Rain, snow, and pain aside, this was a hallmark trip for me. I felt proud of myself and successful. For eight days I was a mountain woman. I felt like I had earned a Girl Scout badge in woodsiness.

Chapter Eleven

Capping

The Capping Ceremony is an endangered species in nursing education. However, County School of Nursing has maintained some archaic traditions that are seldom found in nursing schools today. Capping is a rite of passage that takes place at the end of the first semester. It says you've made it, you are no longer a novice, an outsider. You have served on the front line, you have slept in the trenches. You have earned your cap.

Earning your cap is a mixed blessing. From now on getting dressed in the morning will include pinning a precariously balanced, stiff white hat onto your head. It is the finishing touch on an already absurd uniform. But it is also a symbol, a symbol of what you have achieved, of how hard you have worked. The emotional connections run deep. No two schools have the same cap. The only women to have worn this cap are the ones who have sweated their hearts out in the halls of County.

We who considered ourselves sophisticated played down the upcoming capping ceremony. The men were especially flippant about it. They received pins, not caps. On the whole, nothing about the men's uniforms was as ridiculous as ours. We talked about this ceremony with disdain in our voices, but every single one of us agreed to go through with it. I don't believe any of us would have missed it for the world. Then again, I'm a romantic. Maybe the others weren't secretly touched in their hearts. I know I was. Cool as could be, I couldn't wait to pin that awkward looking cap on my head.

Capping is a ceremony of pride, and for me it was personal. It was such a small accomplishment externally. Celebrating one semester of nursing school hardly seems like something to ring bells about. But bells were exactly what I felt like ringing. I didn't invite any of my family or friends. I don't think I even mentioned it to them. I would have felt ridiculous. There is nothing sophisticated or cool about a capping ceremony.

The younger, less inhibited students were making quite a ruckus over the upcoming event. They invited every person they had ever known. Their parents would be there to take them out to dinner afterward. The thought of my family sitting through a long, silly ceremony, in an auditorium on the main floor of the County hospital, was appalling to me. This was a day to be spent with my cohorts. They were the ones who would understand its importance.

I wanted to go through capping with Michael. He had been beside me through most of first semester. He had left my favorite cookies in my mail box and roses on my door. He taught me fencing and CPR. He massaged me, made love with me, and took me miles away from the county wards. We had held each other in laughter, lust, and tears.

I wanted to be with Evelyn, Susan, and the people in my clinical group. I hadn't told my friends about how much I had hated what I had experienced at County. That had never seemed like an acceptable subject. I have no idea what, if any, internal struggle they may have experienced on the wards. I was proud of them, I was proud of me. I glowed with our accomplishments. It may have been the champagne, it may have been the pot, we all looked pretty radiant that day.

The capping ceremony was to begin around six pm. By mid-morning, I thought evening was never going to come. The air in the dorm was full of festival and party by ten a.m. The voices of the girls had raised to the level of shrieks and shrill laughter. They were as excited and high as horses on a windy morning. By noon the champagne was flowing. Cheap champagne, and lots of it.

Grade B movies and novels have extolled the abilities of student nurses to party hearty. I hate to support stereotypes, especially when I am a member of the group being classified, but student nurses do exhibit a true talent for letting go. They were literally dancing in the halls. I love the sight of females unbridled and at play. When they aren't thinking about how they look, or what men will think of them, women are wonderful. Dancing in their underpants, combing each other's hair, laughing, yelling, swearing. I truly believe women are their most beautiful when there isn't a man around to observe them. Its a shame the men frequently miss the best we have to offer because we're afraid they won't like the view.

All of the women had been told to purchase three uniforms at the beginning of first semester. Admission to County is like joining the army - you learn to obey orders. These dresses had been custom fit to our individual measurements to ensure that they would not fit at all. Upper classmen had passed on the word to the freshmen women to save one uniform until the end of the first semester to wear for Capping. The week before the ceremony was spent making alterations on this pristine uniform. I washed and dried my uniform with four of those fabric softener sheets, trying to kill the super-starched feel of it. I shortened it and tightened it, but it still looked like hell. I had to stand in military position to keep the darts from meeting each other in the center of my chest. This was just as well, as it had a pleasing effect on my posture.

I didn't venture down to the men's floor. I imagine they were doing their own laid back version of the student nurse dance. It would be appealing to think that they were also dancing in their underwear, and helping each other shave.

Finally the hour had arrived, it was time to get Capped. We gathered in the dimly lit corridor of Unit One. This was the same hall we walked down daily to the doctor's cafeteria. It had been altered slightly for the occasion. It was still dim, dingy, and slightly foul smelling, but the usual array of gomers and patients had been cleared out, to make way for the ceremony. Student nurses, faculty, and family members crowded the entrance to the auditorium.

Our first semester Nursing 101 instructors were here to organize and greet us. Each instructor gathered their group and began to give directions. It took awhile to get our attention. We had been distracted by the variety of caps our instructors had earned from their nursing schools. Nurses rarely wear their caps. Wearing caps is reserved for students, fanatics, and for those making a statement. This was my first glimpse of how truly lucky I was in my choice of nursing schools.

Nursing caps range in style from the Nightengalish, to the absurdly comical. Ours was a very crisp, starched, traditional affair with clean lines. It looks like a nurse's cap should look. Nurses in the movies wear this type of cap. I don't know what got into the minds of the people designing caps for some of the schools. I have noted that the schools on the East Coast seem to have a particularly whimsical idea of what belongs on a nurse's head.

The caps are always white; this is a given. From here the guidelines of common sense and gravity have been completely discarded. There were several variations on the dixie cup theme consisting of little pleated white cups, set upside down on a grown woman's head, usually charmingly trimmed with lace. No exaggeration, these caps look like inverted paper nut cups from a bridal shower. It takes a tower of ego and integrity to hold one's head erect while balancing such silliness on top of it.

The miniature mortarboards intrigued me. These caps were designed just like the ones worn by graduating college and high school seniors. Only they were petite and feminine, about six inches across. I assume these caps were intended to signify the scholarly aspects of nursing, but in a dainty, delicate manner.

There are virginal, bridal, overtones in all this capping business. Though unchaste rumors have been circulated about Florence Nightingale, and just how she may have ministered to the troops in the Crimean Wars, there remains a beloved image of nurses as cloistered, nun-like, virginal earth mothers. Nurses are often thought of as never producing their own offspring, but caring for everyone else's. I believe that assuming a nurse has no personal life makes it easier for society to make tremendous demands on her professional life.

Some of our instructors flinched a little as we eyed the doilies on their heads. They looked sheepish and apologetic. But they possessed too much integrity to wear a cap other than the ill-conceived object designed by their alma maters. A misplaced capacity for loyalty can often lead one to bear the unbearable. We kindly kept our hysterics in check. We forced our faces into solemn masks of respect as we observed this imaginative array of headgear. Our faculty was not fooled by our demeanor, but they appreciated our tact.

Not much of the ceremony itself remains in my mind. There were the usual boring speeches made by hyper-achieving students, a guest speaker or two, and a truly forgettable speech given by the Director of the School of Nursing. I don't remember a word she said. To be fair, I don't remember a word any of them said.

I do remember how we received our caps. Each group took it's turn being called to the stage. One by one, our clinical instructor pinned our caps on our heads. This moment was worth sitting through the dull speeches. I was toward the end of our group. With sparkling, loving solemnity, Mrs. Merlin reached up, and pinned a cap on each of our heads and a gold pin on Gregory and John's lapel.

I have a yearbook from my class in nursing school. There are over thirty pictures of our Capping ceremony. It was the most highly represented event of our nursing school experience. So I guess I was not the only one who was affected strongly by that day. One of the pictures is of me, having just received my cap from Mother Merlin. I tower over Helen Merlin by at least six inches. The look on her face is one of surprised joy. Her hands are pulled back in shock. She can't believe the cap has remained in place. I have a look of skeptical hopefulness. I am aware my cap is precariously held to my head by one bobby pin, clinging to a single small pin curl. I must now carefully cross the stage to where another student is waiting in the wings to secure my cap more thoroughly to my head.

The picture is perfect, everything is there; my abomination of a uniform collapsing on my chest, my long neck, with it's muscle tensed, trying to balance the unbalancable. My face is a picture of contained joy. Just visible in the picture is a glimpse of the cowboy pin I wore on my uniform. This was not a legitimate decoration, it was strictly acting out. Each graduating nurse receives a school pin. This is not like the gold-colored job received by the men at capping. This is a fourteen karat gold pin, unique to the school. Most nurses do wear their graduation pin on their uniform. It takes a lot of years and effort to get this pin, and it is rarely taken lightly. The school engraves your initials and the date of your graduation on the back.

As a student nurse, I obviously had no pin. This uniform was demoralizing enough that I didn't see any reason why I should also go pinless. I happened to possess a really neat, painted, tin, cowboy pin. He's a good looking cowboy with steely eyes, a serious mouth, and a red scarf. He's got a green shirt and a blue cowboy hat. I pinned him over my heart, above my left breast. People never acknowledged that I had done this. No one told me to remove the pin, no one ever mentioned it. But I felt better wearing it. I felt like less of a white duck in a row, and more like me. Whenever I put on my uniform, I also put on my pin, even for graduation. Just a small bird, flipped to the world.

Once we were all capped the event came to a ceremonial end. The exact ending I don't recall. I'm even a little fuzzy on the entire following hour. My memory picks up with me feeling like a sardine in a car, definitely filled with too many people. We were on our way to celebrate. Our group included John, Gregory, Sharon, Susan, Michael, Evelyn, and myself. We began by taking ourselves out to an Armenian restaurant for dinner, which I have lost track of all together. The memorable part of the evening for me took place after dinner. I am very sure it was John's idea. He strongly believed we needed to visit the Pleasure Chest.

The Pleasure Chest is a store, in a questionable part of town, that specializes in sexual paraphernalia for those with a taste for the odd. I guess this was a bonding moment for John with the rest of us. Sharon and Gregory appeared rather at home here perhaps they had been privileged with a prior glimpse into John's psyche. For me, the store was a brand new visual bonanza. I had been in one sex shop previously. It was a brightly lit, lime green and apple red, cheery suburban version of a sex shop. It's design was meant to be friendly and open, so as not to frighten the timid. It was the Hallmark version of sex; Debbie Boone could have bought a vibrator there.

Stronger souls than Debbie would have shriveled in the Pleasure Chest. But I'm tough, I can take it. Show me your most bizarre, I'm cool. I feigned an air of casual boredom, as I examined display after display of really strange shit. People are doing weird stuff to each other out there. People are lucky to live through this kind of sex. I've heard some people don't live through it, and I believe it. John never took his eyes off me as I checked out some of his favorite toys. I believe my face was an impenetrable mask of nonchalance. John kept waiting, waiting for my reaction. I was just perverse enough not to give him one. I knew I was the group's token square. Michael was actually much more square than me; he was so out of it he didn't count. John was looking to get a rise out of me. So I casually walked along comparatively shopping leather restraints and chains.

A Boand is a born shopper. Location and item make very little difference; if it has a price tag, we're interested. I can comparison shop bobby sox at K-Mart, or handbags at Neiman's. If goods and money are changing hands, I am in my element. I shifted into my mall mode. I became one with the Pleasure Chest. John couldn't have been happier. A little confused, but happy. He actually had someone who could intelligently discuss which leather restraints were the best buy for the money. He had the best of all worlds, a woman with a frugal, critical eye, willing to examine whips and chains. Sadistic toys have their purchasing charm, but it is limited. Twenty minutes in the Pleasure Chest left me pretty well sated.

When the allure of the Pleasure Chest faded, we began to look for another post-capping activity. The tone for the evening was clearly set. We were spinning our way down into a hole of degradation. This seemed the appropriate counter point to the virginal pomp of capping. We just happened to be ten minutes from another of John and Gregory's favorite spots, the Kit Kat Club. The name is the classiest thing about this joint. We were in a truly terrible part of town. If we got killed here, we would deserve it. The men were juiced; this was gonna be good.

TOTALLY NUDE GIRLS. Why not? I had spent the afternoon watching beautiful girls, draped in dreadful uniforms, stiffly receiving their caps. Why not spend the evening watching plain girls, TOTALLY NUDE, dance? We walked into a morgue of a club. The place was dark, and big enough to have absolutely no charm. Small round tables, large enough to hold a drink, and a single pair of heavily weighted elbows, crowded around the stage. The closest tables were shoved right up against the stage. It must be hell to be a myopic voyeur. The perimeter of the room was lined with green vinyl booths, held almost intact with aging silver tape. We crowded our group into one of these booths. Within moments, from out of the smoky darkness, a cocktail waitress appeared. We ordered our drinks, and waited for the show to begin.

Gregory was of course using a fake I.D. He was so at home here no one would have questioned him anyway. After a long wait, sitting at a slimy wet table, the music finally began. It was some Arabic type piece, supposedly sensual, played on a scratchy record. The woman that plodded gracelessly across the stage looked about thirty-five. She appeared distracted, as if she had just put down her Big Mac and Coke, and hadn't finished chewing yet. She glanced around the room, unenthusiastically eyeing the tiny crowd of about twelve people, including ourselves. With a look of total boredom she began to listlessly move to the music.

This was pathetic. This had the potential to be a real downer. It got worse as she began to remove her scarves to reveal the promised TOTALLY NUDE GIRL. This "girl" was so much better when covered up that it was humiliating. Once she got down to the G-string she began to writhe on the floor on the edge of the stage. Now I saw the purpose for the proximity of the tables. For five bucks you could touch. We were lucky, she decided to let things rest with the g-string. We were spared this TOTALLY NUDE GIRL.

I was more than a little disappointed. This was not the flash and sparkle of striptease dancing that I had fantasized. I was expecting to be teased and entranced by the seductive movements of a beautiful woman slowly, hauntingly, disrobing. This was not titillating; this was depressing. Susan, Evelyn, and Sharon looked as disgusted and bored with the whole thing as I was. These women were not prudes, they just wanted a good show. Now, maybe we should have considered our location. The Kit Kat Club may not be a mecca for strip talent.

John and Gregory seemed to be able to get past our offended sense of aesthetics, and enjoyed the show. They focused on tits and ass and let Siskel and Ebert worry about talent and joy. Michael seemed downright uncomfortable. He would have rather been back at the dorm, wrapped around me. I was beginning to see his point. The night of capping wound down the way many nights of overindulgence do. They come to kind of a slow fizzling end. It was clear there were going to be some interesting bedfellows that night. I wanted to stick around to see who ended up with whom. Michael knew where he planned to end up and was tired of waiting. We said goodbye in front of the others, and then went to our separate rooms. He cleaned up and joined me in a few minutes. We had kept our sexual and romantic involvement private. This was by my choice. I was not offering Michael a monogamous relationship. He knew about Jeff, he knew I might choose to date others. It was a way for me of keeping some balance. County was a small place, and people have the need to categorize things within the scope of their experience and understanding. I did not want the limitations of being labeled as Michael's girlfriend. We had talked about all of this. He was willing to accept my conditions. Michael and I were lovers almost five months, before Susan, my suitemate, even knew.

The night of Capping ended for me quiet and warm. I was happily curled up in my water bed with Michael. Others were happily curled up in other beds, but that is their story, and they can tell it.

Chapter Twelve

The Troll Under The Bridge

Capping was over, first semester, Nursing 101, was behind us. We all felt a little smarter and stronger. We knew the basics of nursing and were ready to move on to some serious stuff. Well, I wasn't so eager to move on to serious blood and guts nursing. I liked learning new skills in the nursing lab. This was greatly preferable to practicing them on real patients. The reality was that the loving, protective wing of Mother Merlin was being abruptly removed . Personally, I felt anxiety about this. Others were not expressing much concern about moving on to a new semester. I figured they were either: a. mute with fear; b. stupidly unaware of the difficulties lying ahead of us; or c. truly eager to get "up close and personal" with the gory intimacies of nursing.

Second semester, Nursing 102, was broken up into three rotations: medical, surgical and orthopedic. The core of our clinic group did not want to separate. We decided to sign up en masse, as a clinic group, for 102. Michael, Evelyn, and Annie-Whammy's best friend Cathleen decided to join our group. The rest of us that chose to stick together included Sharon, Annie-Whammy, Sara, Gregory, John, Maria, and myself.

Cathleen and Annie-Whammy were inseparable and hell on wheels. Their builds were similar, short and chunky. Cathleen struck me with her beauty. Her plump form was topped with a magnificent face. Her lovely smile, sparkling light blue eyes, fair skin, and dark hair belonged on a movie screen.

We had created the perfect group, but the gods who make nursing school decisions were not all sugar and spice. They decided to get even with us for being so presumptuous as to plan our own group, and gave us Muriel Nicholson, R.N. as an instructor. Fate was not smiling the day she created Muriel, in fact Fate may have had a yeast infection that day. Muriel's life seemed not only a blight to Muriel, but to all she touched, and she was about to touch us.

Nicholson was short, fat, mean, and ugly. Ugliness is rarely a case of nasty looking features; there are few truly ugly people. Ugliness is usually a result of some deep, personal dissatisfaction with oneself, reflected outward against the world. Looking at a picture of Nicholson in my yearbook, there is nothing intrinsically unpleasant about her face. Her features could have as easily moved to loving and warm as to mean and nasty. Nastiness and ugliness were her's by choice; a bad choice for her, a worse choice for us.

Our introduction to Nicholson was classic. We walked into the room, and our new instructor said, "I'm your worst nightmare come true." I have heard this statement at least ten times from different instructors, and it always pisses me off for the same reason. I find it presumptuous for some little squat of a person to assume they are my worst nightmare. I can do a hell of a lot better than this in the nightmare division. Nicholson and I were a match born in Hell. It was going to be a long semester.

My worst fear became realized when I learned Nicholson was not bright. Power, in the hands of a simpleton, is my worst nightmare. So the truth is, Nicholson was right, and that really pissed me off. She sat in a small classroom with us, laying down the law. We were her serfs, and she was our feudal lord. She was a slovenly woman, a heavy smoker, with tinted glasses. Her legs were so heavy she frequently sat with her thighs wide apart in the beaver position; thankfully she usually wore pants. She told us her standards were high, she expected excellence, and would be watching us like a hawk. I saw her as a predator waiting for her prey to stumble.

This was Mrs. Nicholson's first semester teaching at County. She had never worked as a County nurse. She had previously taught at a city college. This is a tough way to come to County. Students and faculty frequently look at credentials more critically than the administration might. County nurses are snobs, even the students. They are not too impressed with a junior college nursing program. A nurse who hasn't served his or her time on the wards at County or at an equally tough teaching hospital is viewed with a very critical eye.

There was a fork in her road, just before entering the classroom that first day, where Nicholson could have taken one of several different directions. She could have chosen to befriend us, make us her allies, owned up to her lack of experience. We could all grow together. She could have put up a facade of being all-knowing, but then we might have approached her with tough questions. Instead, Nicholson chose the role of the evil troll under the bridge, and we were stuck playing the frightened children, waiting to be eaten. I believe she came to hate her role as much as we hated ours.

Our clinical group's first rotation was medical on the cardiac unit with Nicholson. This was a mixed blessing for me. Cardiology is a very clean form of medicine. There were no oozing wounds, dripping tubes, or other icky stuff. The patients, however, can be very sick. They may be receiving mixtures of potent medications that require careful monitoring. This was our first time to be responsible for our patients' medications. I was afraid of killing someone. I was afraid of misdosing a patient, and accelerating or decelerating their heart beyond it's ability to cope. This is not just new student jitters. It certainly was jitters, but it was also reality. These medications have the potential to be lethal.

Nicholson managed to make medicating patients an absolute nursing school horror. She loved this. She had found her way to deal with clinic. The medication room on the cardiac ward was large. It had lots of shelves, drawers of meds and one stool. The stool was the deciding factor in Nicholson's fascination with medications. She plopped her big round butt down on that stool and didn't move until break time. Once every twenty minutes she would waddle over to the break room to smoke a cigarette. Other than breaks, Nicholson was parked on that stool. The evil troll had found her ideal spot and set up camp.

There she sat, breath fouled from coffee and cigarettes, waiting for us to come for our medications. She would glow with confidence as a new victim walked into the room. When one gives meds in nursing school, one is required to know a great deal about the patient and the medication. You must know your patient's diagnosis and case history. You must know all meds they are taking, the indications, contraindications, the interactions. You must know what an overdose and a reaction look like. You must know the toxic effects, side effects, preparations, route of administration, dosage, therapeutic uses, the pharmacological properties, and finally how the stuff works. A patient on the cardiology ward may be receiving ten to twelve different medications. This is a shitload of stuff to memorize after you spend hours looking up all the information.

We would go back to the wards after dinner and study our patient's chart to prepare for the next day. We would take notes on the pertinent information, then head to our dorm rooms to look up the details. Inevitably one would overlook a major piece of information, and have to return to the hospital to retrieve it. This was terrific experience. We learned a lot about drugs. We also learned how over-medicated and improperly medicated many of our patients were. We frequently studied the charts more intently than the intern on the case, who probably saw fifteen patients to our one. I caught many medication errors on patients' charts while working at County. My experience was not unique; it was universal. I would spend an evening hunting down the intern with my drug textbook, and my patient's chart in hand.

Interns would vary in their response to my approaching them to discuss a case. The hunky Joe Cools would smile warmly, put an arm around me, and cozy up for a profound discussion of the case. The smarter-than-thou types would, for a patronizing moment, give me a few precious seconds of their time. The terrific interns, in who's care I hope to land if I ever need them, would sit down to discuss the case with a peer. Whatever their initial response, I would have their attention once I started pointing out medication errors, and, for the slower intern, the implication of these errors.

Usually interns were grateful for the information. They always acted on it, because they knew I would be pointing it out to someone else if they didn't. It was interesting to note how the interaction would go once I pointed out the error. Super Cools dropped me like a hot potato, smarter-than-thous avoided me like a social disease, and terrific interns became my cohorts and friends.

The next morning, I, along with the rest of my group, would show up for clinic with notes in hand. We would cram till the very last second before entering the medication room. Eventually, I would have to enter and face Nicholson, in order to medicate my patient. I would give a weak, forced smile, and begin to search for the medications I needed. She would drill me on my meds, I would sputter out my answers. My anxiety was so high, I was ready to hand a patient a rectal suppository to swallow. Nicholson nearly died of joy pointing this out to me.

It might have been worth it if she had died of joy. At least she would have gone happily, and we would have been rid of her. No such luck, she survived this delightful moment, to experience yet another, at someone else's expense. There were a couple of secrets we were to learn in dealing with Nicholson. First, the woman really was not bright, or well educated. There were only a few medications she knew well, silly little meds like Doss, a stool softener. That's where she would catch you. While you were explaining the intricacies of diuretics and sympathomimetics, she would distract you and say "tell me what you know about Doss". This was unbelievable. Everybody on the unit was on this drug. "It makes your shit soft, what do you want to know?"

She wanted to know the action of Doss. Somewhere, somehow, she had managed to learn and retain the action of this stool softener on the sigmoid colon, and she was lording it over us like the secret to the universe. This is not tough information to access. We looked up the action of Doss, and passed it around the group. We all now knew as much about medications as Nicholson did. From there on out it was just a matter of confidence and maintaining a poker face. Nicholson didn't know what we were talking about. As long as we spoke in large technical words, she was confused. She would respond in a gruff manner, "fine, but make sure you read the labels." This is probably the best advice you can give anyone about administering medications anyway; total traumatization was not necessary. I never forgave her for the pain and indignities I suffered at her hand. To me she remains the evil troll under the bridge. It was a pleasure to be free from Nicholson's grasp and to move on to an instructor with a gentler touch.

Chapter Thirteen

It Only Takes A Five To Pass

Grades are not important. Everyone knows this. An "A" student is not an intrinsically finer person than a "B" student. Theoretically, you do not compete among your classmates for grades, you only try to do your best. What matters is what you learn, not the score you receive. There are hundreds of these uplifting sayings regarding grades. These sayings have one purpose, to console those receiving less than an "A". Other than that, they don't mean shit, and anyone receiving an "A", knows this. An "A" always looks nicer than a "B". It may be a matter of culturally induced aesthetics, but I've never met anyone yet who preferred the look of a "B" to an "A" on the top of an exam paper.

All grades at County were filtered down to the students via their mail boxes. Commuters and dorm dwellers alike were assigned a mail box in the dorm lobby. Those of us who lived in the dorms checked our boxes every time we passed them. Some days I would check my mail box ten to twelve times out of habit. At any hour of the day something might be placed in my box. Intermittent positive reinforcement is the best way to insure consistent behavior. We were better trained than Pavlov's dogs. It would have caused me physical pain to walk past my box without looking in it. Understanding our fixation with our mail boxes, we took advantage of this form of communication. This is where Michael frequently left me cookies. This was the place to receive obscene notes, sarcastic comments, small packages, U.S. mail, and grades.

You could tell who had recently had an exam by their approach to the mail boxes. People varied on their post-exam approach. Mine was a determined march up to the mail box. I had tried early in my nursing career to master a casual post-exam stroll. My stress level had been too high. There was a touch too much rush in my approach to qualify as a stroll. Evelyn went beyond stroll. Her approach was so slow, imperious, and disdainful, one got the impression she was passing judgment on her instructors, rather than the reverse. The men appeared less creative than the women. They had one basic move, awesome indifference. "Hey, I don't care man, fuck grades." I have noticed that males under stress, or in pain, often rely on very basic forms of communication.

Grades are not important. Everyone knows this. So the first thing out of everyone's mouth is "what'd ya get?" The very act of inserting a key in a lock would elicit this articulate remark from at least ten mouths. The County grading system was based on a nine point scale. A nine was an "A", eight was an "A-", or a "B+", based on your point of view. Seven was a "B". The important number was a five. Five was a "C", and a passing grade. Below five was not considered passing. From here down it was just a matter of how far below passing you were.

Nursing classes had to be taken sequentially. If you failed a class, you had to drop out, retake the class and pass it, before you could proceed to the next term. Passing became imperative. Our eloquent men came through with a soothing slogan, "it only takes a five to pass". Of course this slogan was soothing only if you scored a five or better. In the case of a four or less, one had to fall back on "fuck grades".

My grades at County were fairly typical of my college career. I received mostly "B"s, a few "C"s, and some "A"s. I am not a dedicated student. This is a strange statement coming from someone with twelve years of college and graduate education. I am the most over-educated non-student I know. My approach to school has always been casual. Maybe this is why I have been able to tolerate so much of it. I spend very little time studying or reading text books. I generally read novels. I would learn the material by attending lecture and taking excellent notes. Usually, I only have to read through my notes once or twice and I have all the important information from lecture. As long as the material is theoretical, abstract, or conceptual, I am in good shape. I get "A"s in this type of class. It's the classes that require memorization that kill me. Nursing does not require a great deal of rote memory, so I was not in bad shape. Learning neuroanatomy to get my doctorate nearly wiped me out.

The most frequent grade in my mail box was a seven. A seven is ok. It's nothing to write home about, but I was in no danger of failing. I did receive an occasional five. This is when I was thankful to have such a comforting slogan to fall back on. I would shrug, my hopes deflated and quote, "well, it only takes a five to pass." Good friends who were quick on the draw would usually step in and say this for you, thus demonstrating their participation in the group deception that grades were not important.

I dreaded these post-test gatherings around the mail boxes. Generally I only dreaded them when I knew my grade was iffy. If I knew I had aced an exam, I would storm to the box, rush it open, and dig in for my grade. Occasionally a terrible surprise comes this way. More than a few times I have torn open the folded sheet of paper to view my nine, only to be shocked by a seven or less. These were lousy moments. I would be surrounded by a dozen mouths all forming the words at once, "what'd ya get?" Disappointment is an emotion I hate displaying publicly. It's not as bad as humiliation or devastation, but it's still unsightly, and I loathe it. I would fold to the social pressure of the group's need to know, and announce my grade. I would do this unless my grade was less than a five. I only received a couple of grades this low and I was always aware I had not done well on the test. In these cases, I would wait to get my grade until the entire lobby was abandoned, and then discreetly approach my mail box.

There are always the students who hang in there at a five, struggling along. The six delights them, a four depresses them, and they have seen more threes, twos, and ones, than they care to admit. These are the ones to whom failure is a real possibility. What surprises me is that they are so much more resolute about it than I would be. They are rarely panicky, sweating or crazy. Their approach is more often quiet, accepting, and exhausted. Often these have been friends of mine, not one of my close friends, but people on the periphery of my life. They are people who study long hours, taking in tremendous amounts of information, and getting it all jumbled up in the process. It frustrates me tremendously. I want to take control of their lives. I want to give them my notes, and say, "study these and nothing else". Ask no questions that can't be answered by what is in my notes. In the case of studying, less is often more. I want to trim out all the fat for them, and just show them what they need to know.

Some brains are of the type that, when handed a pile of information, they immediately sort out what is important and what is not. My mind works this way. It tosses out the peripheral crap before I am even aware that I've heard it. I have seen other types of minds work. Some are compelled to assimilate every piece of information thrown their way. It requires the intellect of a genius to sort out the intake with this type of mind. I am lucky, I have a mind that makes learning easier. We are all gifted in unique ways. Whenever one of my gifts gives me a natural advantage I feel guilty. I used to feel tremendously guilty. I have come to understand others will have gifts that I don't have. It is just a matter of the hand we are dealt, and guilt is a useless response.

I am currently in the process of learning to weed out useless responses from my repertoire. However, while in nursing school, they were a staple of my emotional diet. I would stand at my mailbox, eyeing my easily achieved eight, and feel terrible guilt as some sincere student pulled out a hard won five. I would then compound guilt with idiocy by saying, "it only takes a five to pass." No one smacked me for this. They all knew I was trying to be kind and uplifting. I felt like smacking myself for being an asshole. We all secretly know grades do mean shit, and everybody wants an "A". We want the "A's" because they are validating. An "A" says you're smart, you know your stuff, you did a good job. A "D" or an "F" says you're a dopehead and ought to be bounced off the planet. Personally, I couldn't take the latter. I felt my right to be on this planet was too tenuous to risk an official stamp of disapproval.

Evelyn and Susan both made slightly better grades than I did. They hung in there in the "A-" to "B+" range. They both graduated with some level of honors. Evelyn and Susan studied. They weren't hounds about it, but plenty of times they couldn't play. They wanted to study. This was a foreign concept to me. I have never preferred study to play. For this I have often been called a bad influence. I took a very logical approach to studying. I could study four hours for an exam and probably score an eight or a nine, or I could review my notes for forty-five minutes and probably score a seven. With good luck, on this second method, I would get an eight or even a nine; with bad luck I would get a six. I was willing to play the odds knowing chances were I would get a seven. I like "A"s, I just wasn't willing to give up play time to get an inordinate number of them.

What about learning for the joy of acquiring knowledge? That my brain does constantly. To be alive, is to be learning. Learning the convolutions of my psyche and of those I love, figuring out what is going on with the world as I perceive it, is the learning I live for. Unfortunately, no one has offered to pay me for this wealth of knowledge. My father taught me early that if no one will pay you for it, it isn't worth anything. But my father has lied to himself and to me about this, and I know it. He told me this to instill a sense of financial worth. Regarding the external world he holds this true. I got confused and thought I must value my gifts and skills by his rule of ecconomics. The result was I scored myself rather low on the value scale. In reality, my father treasures deeply many things for which the world wouldn't pay him a cent, and one of them is me. I know this by the way he holds my hand, caresses me, and loves me. If I had payed more attention to his actions, and less to his words, I would have come out with clearer thinking on the subject of me.

Though I didn't require A's of myself I did not want to fail. I have a method for studying; most students do. Seventy-two hours before an exam, I begin to think about it. I realize that three days is way too far ahead to study for any test. I release myself from the thought and go play. Forty-eight hours before an exam I begin to take it more seriously. I examine carefully the study hours I have available to me; I may even write them down for a particularly tough test. I then acknowledge I can't possibly study for two days straight. I will need at least some breaks and relaxation periods. I decide to relax now to get that over with so I can concentrate on studying without interruption. At this point the number of people available to play with me is beginning to dwindle. Usually I could find some other soul who was into avoidance that I could lure to a movie. In the twenty-four hours preceding an exam the pressure is on. If I wanted a companion in procrastination I had to be selective. No one would come play with me with just gentle nudging at this time. I must be aggressive, pushy, even insulting. I must bring into question a person's ethics and value system in order to coerce them into play.

Tactics such as these require some sense of responsibility. It would be morally reprehensible for me to seduce a student in danger of failing away from studying. I had a small select group I felt free to hit on in this manner. Their grades were better than mine, and they had strong enough defenses to ignore my insults, if they were determined to study. People didn't get angry at my aggressive behavior. They recognized it as my pre-test pattern and told me to "bug off". Persistence does pay off. Occasionally I would get lucky and find someone as bored with this test business as I was. Usually though I was left to my own devices. I have found shopping to be an excellent way to spend the six hours preceding the very last possible study moment.

The last possible study moment for me is seven-thirty p.m. the evening before a morning exam. The last possible study moment for any test taking place after nine a.m., is one hour before the exam. I am a morning person. I can't possibly study after eight-thirty at night, my brain is too sleepy. The first thing in the morning my brain is too hungry, I must have food.

I know my situation is not unique. I have listened to others describe study patterns very similar to mine. Some clinical psychologists who specialize in effective study methods (an incredibly boring group of people) have charts depicting people like me. They show stick figures walking to and from Coke machines, watching T.V., and staring out the window, with their circular heads in their little stick hands. The face on these figures is always a big, round, unhappy face. On the contrary the good stick figure, with it's book in hand, is sporting a big smiling happy face. I have always considered the guys holding up these charts to be the biggest ninnies I have ever seen.

Chapter Fourteen

The Queen of Psychosocial Nursing

A wonderful new term, psychosocial, had evolved in nursing prior to my entering the profession. The psychosocial aspect of patient care focuses on the patient's psychological and social needs. The idea was to consider the impact of disease on the patient's emotional and personal life. I am an emotional sponge. I absorb and internalize other people's emotions like a Handy-Wipe sops up milk. This trait can be disabling for me in my relations with those I love, but it made me one hot psychosocial nurse.

The psychosocial concept in nursing saved my ass, and made life on the wards bearable. I first learned about this phrase during second term. This was the term when we were required to begin writing care plans. Care plans are the pits. I have no idea whether or not they are still in vogue.

The title is self-explanatory. Care plans are long, drawn out, detailed descriptions of how a nurse plans to care for a patient. Like many things, in theory the idea is not bad. It is an idea conceived by the mind of an academic, tenaciously latched onto by an administrator, and thrust upon a practitioner. It is an idea that looks beautiful on paper, sells well to the brass, and to work with it is totally impractical. Wonderfully elaborate plans, delineating the minutiae of a patient's care, beautifully written up on over-sized graph paper, usually in full color, were the way to an instructor's heart. They were also the way to a good grade in a clinical course.

Once on the hospital unit, the fantasy plan was usually tossed aside, and the realities of nursing at County took precedence. Care plans really were a pain. Done well, they required hours of research on diseases, medications, treatments, prognosis, and home care follow-up. The one saving grace about care plans was the term psychosocial. The psychosocial needs of the patient made up the last topic to be covered on the care plan. I loved this concept. I had enthusiasm for it. I was alone in my joy of psychosocial nursing; everyone else thought it sucked. I became the Queen of Psychosocial Nursing, and my patients loved me for it.

I found that dealing with this psychosocial stuff was not the thing for which most doctors and nurses have the time or the inclination. I would make the time, because it was the only aspect of nursing that really gave me joy. I don't want to know the physiological implications of someone's illness. I want to know how they feel about it. How does their spouse feel about it? What's going on with their kids through all of this?

As I moved through my chores, I would explore with my patients the details of their experiences while ill. While I attended to their physical needs I would listen, discerning any emotional needs where I might be of assistance. This wasn't because I was an all-caring angel out to heal the aching hearts of the ill. I focused on my patients' emotions because this was an area with which I was comfortable. I will gravitate to laughter and tears over blood and guts every time. The hospital was full of people happy to deal with blood and guts, and a little short on those who could cope with tears.

Our clinical group was now beginning the middle rotation of Nursing 102. After Murial Nicholson's reign of terror we were all a little nervous about facing our next instructor, Catherine Miller, for our surgical experience. Catherine is an intelligent woman, with a serious, competent nature. Nicholson had set my confidence back severely. Catherine was a more recently educated nurse. A beautifully written care plan gave her a warm glow. She saw attending to the psychological needs of a patient as the new wave in nursing. This was a semester where I was going to be able to shine.

Mrs. Miller liked to assign one patient for us to work with for the entire week (by this time we were spending three full days a week on the wards). I was either looking competent or terribly in need of a challenge, because my first week Catherine assigned me Mr. Kabakian. He was a fifty-five year old Armenian, with a wife and three young children. He was also a very sick man.

On paper, Mr. Kabakian did not look good. He had six tubes or drains going in or out of him. He had undergone surgery to remove stones from his gall bladder. Things had not gone smoothly. Mr. Kabakian now had a hospital induced pseudomonas infection at the site of his surgery. Pseudomonas is a bacterial infection usually acquired in the hospital due to inadequate hand washing by the staff. This is not an extremely unusual occurrence. The medical profession has incorporated these concepts into it's language. If you go to the hospital and catch an infection, it is a nosocomial infection or disease. If your doctor goofs up and makes you sick or sicker, you now have an iatrogenic disease. If one is so unlucky as to have something like this befall them, its nice to know there are official terms for it.

I sat down and began studying Mr. Kabakian's chart. I worked making notes of all the information I would have to research. His list of medications was endless. The description of all the tubes entering and exiting his body was horrifying. I couldn't believe Catherine had done this to me. I felt like the ultimate victim. I think I felt more sorry for myself than I did for Mr. Kabakian. This was our first day on the surgical unit with Mrs. Miller. We were not working with patients today. We were being oriented to the unit and receiving our patient assignments for the following week. I had looked at the chart and lamented as long as I could I finally went in to meet my patient.

Mr. Kabakian was a big, strong man. He spoke broken English, with a heavy accent. He had a warm, sincere face. He welcomed me with an apologetic smile. I told him I was going to be taking care of him next week. He apologized for the difficulty he knew he would be for me. I immediately lied, and I lied beautifully. My mother would have been proud. "You're no trouble Mr. Kabakian, I am delighted to work with you. I'll look forward to seeing you on Monday."

It wasn't such a big lie, because once I had met him and spoken to him, it was impossible not to care for Mr. Kabakian and his plight. I went home and began the care plan of the century. We had to turn in one major care plan each semester, covering nearly the entire life and times of our patients. The other care plans were more abbreviated versions, slightly more realistic as to might be done on the wards. I had the perfect patient for a massive, four color, with graphics, care plan. His physical problems ranked in the dozens. His care and treatment needs went on and on. I even drew front and back diagrams indicating the entrance or exit of all of his tubes. It would take several days working with Mr. Kabakian to assess his psychosocial needs. But having written him up on paper, my patient was less intimidating. I was ready to work with him face to face.

Monday morning I woke up anxious. I was concerned about working with Mr. Kabakian. I was afraid he was too sick for me to deal with emotionally. By the time I began to wash my face, my anxiety had advanced to pure dread. The man beautifully written up on paper began to fade. He was replaced by the reality of Mr. Kabakian in the flesh. Stoma fear had gripped me around the throat and was squeezing off my air. A stoma is an artificial opening, surgically created, forming a passageway from the inside of the body to the outside of the body, to provide drainage.

My stoma fear is so intense that just describing one causes me to freeze up. I will try to be clear. The type of stoma Mr. Kabakian had was a colostomy. The surgeon takes a loop of bowel, severs it, and brings the end up through an opening in the abdominal skin. The patient's excretory functions then take place through this opening. Sometimes colostomies are temporary and are later surgically reversed. Other colostomies are permanent. People with permanent colostomies learn to care for themselves, and lead normal lives with some dietary changes. People with colostomies are out there among us functioning well; the human being adapts, and life goes on.

I am a queazy nurse. I hate blood and guts. I hate things that ooze. I hate physical trauma and ravaged bodies. One might question my choice of professions given this state of innate repulsions. I didn't. I rationalized this away. I figured there must be some form of clean nursing, where my warm smile and psychosocial skills would be of value. I would eventually find such a haven in nursing, but I had to work my way there via surgery, infected orthopedics, and neurosurgery - some of the drippiest, ooziest, most tube filled places around.

I needed to get my focus off my dread. Self-delusion was the method I usually chose to escape fear or dread. If I didn't have time to work up a good delusion, or if in the rare instance delusion was impossible, then I would make do with diversion. Diversion is a limited tool in dealing with unpleasant thoughts or feelings. I can only divert myself for a short time. Self-delusion, on the other hand, can endure. I personally can sustain a well developed delusion for years.

It was six a.m. Monday morning. I had to be on the unit in one hour, there was no time for delusion. I moved instinctively to diversion. Make-up is a great diversion for me, it ranks right up there with the comic pages. I most frequently used a combination of make-up and the comics to waylay my pre-test panic. I walked into a test smiling and looking great. A mixture of Trudeau, Larson and Lancome would eclipse my fear of impending doom. I have found out later that my fellow students have been very intimidated by my relaxed appearance at tests. They have mistaken my diversionary behavior as a sign of confidence and brilliance.

I had to be careful about my timing. This is always the catch in using diversion to escape fear. I tend to run almost late for most things. I view this as being exactly on time while others have seen this as tardiness. If I get too lost in my diversion I can forget exactly where I have to be, and when. At this point, diversion backfires, and anxiety amplifies times one hundred. I am now late and rushing to something I loathe, which will be even worse for me because I am late. So I watched the clock constantly while applying stunning but subtle make-up. I wanted just enough time to have breakfast and read the comics before walking onto the wards.

I had dawdled around at breakfast long enough that I had to rush directly to the unit. I fooled around with the charts and nursing supplies for as long as possible while screwing up my courage. After fifteen minutes on the unit I had exhausted all legitimate excuses for delaying greeting Mr. Kabakian. I found him propped up against his pillows eating his breakfast. Patient food at County has a standard, processed, sealed-in-plastic-smell. The smell of the food was a little bit noxious, but I was used to it by now. I was not used to the smell of a pseudomonas infection. The sweet, thick smell met me within moments of saying hello to Mr. Kabakian. I have a keen sense of smell, and I have always reacted strongly to unpleasant ones.

I forbade my face to grimace, or my body to recoil. I chatted with Mr. Kabakian while he ate, and I looked him over to make sure there were no obvious problems that needed immediate attention. I glanced around to see if things that were supposed to be flowing in or out of tubes were moving along as they should. He had already washed up, so I collected the linen to change his bed as soon as he finished breakfast.

While Mr. Kabakian was loaded with tubes, they were all attached to bags on poles, with wheels, so he was somewhat mobile. He sat in a chair beside the bed and talked to me while I worked. His sheets were soiled from his oozing wounds. I quickly wound them into a ball and stuffed them into a pillow case. I spread the clean sheets out on the bed. The difference was not lost on him. Mr. Kabakian told me he hated the smell of his infection. The smell disgusted and embarrassed him so much that he hated to have other people around him. He was afraid the doctors, nurses, and his wife would find him disgusting. The thought of his wife being repulsed almost moved him to tears.

I understood; the stench was nearly gagging me. But my physical response was overshadowed by the creative challenge this smell presented. My mind kicked into gear, my patient clearly had a major psychosocial need. Psychosocial Queen came surging forward. I would solve this problem for Mr. Kabakian. I may not be the finest technical nurse he ever saw, but I would make him smell better. Odor control flashed across the screen of my mind. My brain sorted through possible solutions instantly. I thought of a little bottle I had seen somewhere in the hospital. Odor-No, two drops kills any odor for eight hours. Perfect; where did I see this stuff?

It took me a few minutes to remember the ward and the location where I had seen Odor-No. I located several bottles on another unit and nabbed one for Mr. Kabakian. I returned to his room armed with the bottle and several packages of four by four cotton swabs. The way this stuff was supposed to work was you put some on a cloth surface, and it would absorb all odors in an area of approximately six to ten feet. I explained this to Mr. Kabakian while I put several drops on a piece of gauze. I taped the four by four above his bed, waited a moment and took a deep breath. Amazingly, the stuff worked. It absorbed the smell. Mr. Kabakian smelled like he was sitting in the middle of a pine forest after a rain. We both shook our heads, looked at each other and smiled. We hadn't believed it would work. Finally, Mr. Kabakian said, "I smell wonderful".

We were on a roll, Mr. Kabakian and I. He had shared his fears with me, and now that he smelled good, life was getting better. We were both excited. I had my first success with an intimidatingly difficult patient. So what's next, what else bothers you? Mr. Kabakian couldn't believe his good fortune. He had an eager ear attached to a creative problem-solving mind totally dedicated to finding solutions to his needs. He told me he was very unhappy because he had not seen his children in several weeks. He felt isolated from his family, his children were very small, and he was afraid he might die without seeing them again.

This struck me as bizarre. Why hadn't he seen his children? I was still unaware of some hospital rules. Children under twelve were not allowed on many of the units, surgery being one of these. It really frustrated me that I could come up with no immediate solutions. Now that he smelled better Mr. Kabakian wanted to see his children. I worked over this puzzle like a Rubic's Cube, determined to find a solution.

All this psychosocial nursing allowed me to focus away from draining wounds, colostomies, and dressing changes. These things still had to be looked after, but I could think about the real problems, while doing the physical labor. My mind was fully occupied until it was time for lunch. For me, few things take precedence over food.

I left the unit for lunch at the student nurses' cafeteria. Lunch was the only meal that we ate in this room. There was little to get excited about regarding lunch. The broccoli soup was usually edible. After sharing a meal with my friends it was time to get back to the uint and Mr. Kabakian.

County elevators are slow, so slow one might as well use the stairs, especially if you are in a hurry. Since I regularly ran almost late, I was usually in too much of a hurry to take the elevators to the wards. I would most often resort to storming up the stairs, arriving damp, breathless, and flushed, but just on time. I never wanted to dawdle leaving the wards, so I always took the stairs down after work.

The only noticeable thing about lunch today was that I finished faster than usual. I had an extra two or three minutes to spare. This meant I could afford the luxury of taking the elevator. Nothing too special about County elevators, they creak and squeak, stall and moan, smell like a hundred men have watched the Super Bowl in them, and threaten to freeze up altogether mid-ride. Still, this is preferable to a four flight jog after lunch.

The elevator came to a creaky stop, and the doors opened on the fourth floor. I was doing well, only one minute late. The elevator was located in a large corridor. This was a rectangular space, with long halls leading off to either side. The surgery unit was to the left. I had always entered the unit by the side stairway. I had never noticed that outside the main entry doors there were two benches. The benches were obviously for visitors. Frequently staff and visitors have very different impressions of large institutions. I had never noticed the facilities set up for visitors near the entrance to the unit. My oversight was not tremendous. The facilities consisted of two benches still it indicated to me that visits took place just outside the doors of the unit.

In retrospect, it does not surprise me that I was unaware of a visitors facility right outside of our unit. It is a form of self-defense to be able to walk around in an emotional mine field without seeing the constant trauma. Pain was all around us. Therefore, I acquired this skill early at County, as did everyone I knew. I returned from lunch triumphant. I had found a solution for Mr. Kabakian. His wife could bring the children here to visit and he could come out to sit with them by the elevators. Mr. Kabakian was less excited than I was; he had some problems with this plan. The problems all turned out to be ones of esthetics. He didn't like that his hospital gown flapped open in the back and showed his bare ass, who would? Odor-No was effective near his bed, but would it do for travel? How would he conceal his wounds oozing onto his gown? He wanted to see his children, but he didn't want them to see him looking bad.

My parents have trained me well in the importance of looking good. They thought that good grooming will take you even farther than lots of money. I hope this is so, since my skills at grooming far outweigh my skills for obtaining money. I told Mr. Kabakian not to worry, I could make him look and smell good. He believed me. I helped him to the pay phone (no private, in room phones at County) where he called his wife and set up a family visit for two days from now, when I would next be on the unit.

I spent little time thinking about Mr. Kabakian's draining stoma and colostomy. I figured out what I would need to do to freshen him up, and let the rest of the staff worry about his electrolyte levels. I decided this is what is meant by the idea of a team approach to nursing care. I was the psychosocial part of Mr. Kabakian's team.

Wednesday morning I worked to get all of Mr. Kabakian's normal care finished and out of the way. Drains were cleaned, bags were emptied, and contents were measured. All the really ickiest stuff was done that morning to leave the afternoon free. After lunch I collected a fresh gown, towels, safety pins, a razor, and a basin of hot water. I set Mr. Kabakian up so he could shave, changed his dressings, and gave him the clean gown to wear. He stood modeling the gown for me while I pinned the back, hiding tubes and buttocks. I carefully pinned a small cotton square containing two drops of Odor-No onto the inside of his gown. We had to wait until the last minute in our preparations and then move quickly. I figured Mr. Kabakian had about thirty minutes before his clean dressing would be saturated and leak through onto his gown.

My charge was prepared for his party. At the designated time we strolled out to the waiting area. It was a slow stroll. Mr. Kabakian was in pain and moving delicately. I was carefully navigating his two I.V. poles hung with bags and bottles, trying to keep the lines from tangling or dislodging. They were all there waiting for him; his wife, his three children, and a few assorted relatives. I settled him on the bench, arranged his plumbing, and said good-bye. We had planned that I would leave him alone with his family for twenty-five minutes, and then come back to collect him.

Twenty-five minutes later Mr. Kabakian looked tired, happy, and tearful. I knew he was in pain as I helped him up and prepared him for the walk back to bed. His wife was smiling in her tears as she thanked me. There was no pain on the children's faces, they were dancing happily around their father. But the adults knew the pain and suffering Mr. Kabakian endured to see his children. He was a very sick man. This was the first time I admitted to myself that he might not leave the hospital. I was standing in the middle of the pain, the tears, the love, and the loss. I had lost my professional perspective. I had joined the group of people facing the potential pain and loss of dear Mr. Kabakian.

The walk back to his bed was even slower than our earlier walk. He told me how his children looked as if they had grown since he last saw them. He was happy. He got into bed exhausted, ready to sleep. For the first time in my nursing career, I stepped into the linen closet and cried.

Chapter Fifteen

Lost In The Joy Of Romance

Some people innately know how to romance, and others never quite get the hang of it. Those who are not naturals at it generally have to rely on a calculated approach. Michael was about a seven on a one to ten scale of romantic aptitude. My past is checkered with men who usually scored around a three on this scale. I felt fortunate to be the recipient of Michael's romantic skills.

Three months had passed and we were still not public about our relationship. I had finally let Susan and Evelyn in on the details. Other than that, we stayed somewhat discreet for another few months. It was because we were not planning a future together that we kept our romance private. Michael and I had discussed our disparate values and had no intention of getting married. Our classmates knew we were close friends, they just weren't sure how close. Keeping our romance a secret was a pain in the neck, but it also provided us with some scintillating rushes. Nothing rushes the heart, the brain, and the hormones, like an illicit affair. Faster than speed, more compelling than coke, there is nothing like the heat of passion in concealed corridors to distract oneself from the daily conflicts of life.

Romances are like giant pandas, they require very special diets and environments to survive. I had not made any conscious study of romance - I was winging it. A lifelong saturation of movies starring Doris Day, Audrey Hepburn and Katherine Hepburn made up my picture of the perfect romance. I wanted a man who would love me boundlessly and find my gravest imperfections charming beyond comparison. I imagined a man who's face would light up like the morning sun every time I appeared. I wanted him to find me brilliant, warm, funny, beautiful, sexy, compelling, and intriguing. I wanted my prince to be a mirror able to show me all the wonders of me that I couldn't see for myself.

Without ever having experienced it, I instinctively knew how wonderful this would feel. I attempted to play the role of the all seeing mirror for those I loved. Not that I found Michael's every thought charming, or even indicative of clear thinking. But I did carry my Pollyanna attitude forward into our relationship. I focused on the best in Michael. Every wonderful thing I discovered about Michael, I shared with him immediately. I quietly kept to myself all the bad news. I never said, "I hate your politics, the way you dress drives me nuts, I can't stand that you are so much more of a nerd than I am". I wasn't just dishonest with Michael. I wouldn't admit to myself that there were areas of Michael I found disenchanting. I was engaging in a full romance, and only half a relationship.

There is an intrinsic problem with my mirror approach to romance. It has taken me years to sort this out. I believe the catch lies for me in my need to respect and value my mirror. If my prince tells me all the wonders he sees in me (all the wonders I can not see for myself) then I believe the mirror must be cracked. If my prince sees so much in me that I do not, his vision must be clouded. Damn, my mirror is broken, I need a new one. This is not conducive to long term relationships. However, the joy of finding a bright new mirror, shining with enthusiasm for me, did not encourage me to critically examine my premise.

    I have a friend from college who's parents have an artistic flare for labeling her behavior. Her father once told her, "Carolyn, you think with your gonads". Her mother has announced in distress, "Carolyn, you are relationship hopping." These statements were made years apart. Both hit me profoundly. Originally my only concern was how devastated I would have been if my parents had addressed my life so bluntly. Later, I thought about how much Carolyn and I have in common. Currently, I have come to see her parents as articulate wonders, addressing the nature of romance and relationships as we have learned it in the movies. Relationship hopping while thinking with one's gonads; that rather says it all.

    I don't really believe gonads and hormones say it all, but I do think they are a part of it. Hormones, on the whole, are not highly connected to clarity of thought. One thing I have learned about romance is that it is not the place to pursue the search for strength, courage, insight, and honesty. These things create a hostile environment for romance. Not love, it is nurtured by these things, but love is something best done from a position of internal strength. Romance is delicate, it flourishes best when handled gently. The buffered statement, softly spoken and gently worded is how one feeds a romance. Little subtle hints, innuendoes as to what might please one, carefully worded suggestions, are the One-A-Day vitamins of romance.

    I felt tremendously blessed that Michael wanted to have a romance with me. As his shell opened, his warm, joyful, giving nature spilled out and surrounded us both. This was a gift from the gods. This was pure luck. I was not going to mess with this by introducing excessive honesty. If this man could work up romantic feelings for me in the face of my blunt approach, I could release myself from pursuing the touchy issues. I wasn't really ready to pursue strength, courage, insight, and honesty. I was ready to get lost in the joy of romance. So that is what we did. We wrapped our arms around each other. We stared into each other's eyes. We laughed, and played, and made love. We dipped into that warm, dark, intoxicating pool of romance, and took a brief swim.

    Every romance is different and has it's own flavor. Michael and I had a kind of Mutt and Jeff look. We were both uncommon dressers. I would best describe my clothes as stylish, eclectic, and offbeat, sometimes good, sometimes odd. I am not sure how to describe Michael's style. Unlike many men who have no desire to make a fashion statement, Michael was trying to say something. I never figured out just what that message was. Unfortunately, he had not yet discovered natural fibers. His closet was heavily laden with late sixties-early seventies white elephants. Polyester was the dominate fabric for his shirts. He was also fond of hats, and a floor length burgundy wool cape.

How do you tell a man who takes great pride in his look that you think it needs work? Directly, honestly, and lovingly, of course. Luckily or not for the people in my life now, that's mostly what I do. This takes courage though, and an openness to explore the implications of one's own closet. The courage required was not just the willingness to be open and possibly face Michael's irritation. It required that I face the possibility of losing Michael, and that was not something I was willing to do. So, at five feet eight inches, I would put on my high heeled cowboy boots, cashmere sweater, skin tight blue jeans, and walk with long legged strides, next to Michael, five feet four inches, in his polyester shirt, felt fedora hat, and floor length wool cape.

We were an affectionate team of "one does and one doesn't." I danced, Michael didn't, he could scuba dive, I couldn't. I had enough money for the occasional dinner out, Michael didn't. He was health conscious and carried a small vial of bran to sprinkle on his food whenever he ate. I am indulgent, my genetics allow for this. I stay thin while heaping ice cream into my chocolate milk. Michael read science fiction and fantasy novels. I read Ayn Rand, Doris Lessing, and Aldous Huxley. Michael loved backpacking, I loved the tea room at Bullocks department store. Michael was a volunteer, a helper, and altruistic. I am an egotist. I believe most altruistic acts are done to meet one's own needs. On paper, someone like Michael comes out looking much more socially acceptable than I do.

We did have many things in common. Nursing school, especially our experiences on the wards at County, provided a strong bond. We also had friends in common. Michael was considered somewhat out of it by the cooler men on the fourth floor. I'm not sure what the cool guys thought of me. But Evelyn, Gregory, and Susan all liked me, and they were in the center of what's hot. What's hot was determined by what went on, on the fourth floor, where the men lived. County is located on the East side of town, in the barrio. Quick to pick up on the social implications of our location, the fourth floor became Quatro Flats, a bastardization of Steinbeck's **Tortilla Flats**. If you wanted to party, cruise, or hang out, you did it on Quatro Flats. Barrio slang became the vocabulary of the day. This turned out to be helpful. An adequate slang vocabulary cuts through a lot of crap in dealing with adolescent patients. Adolescent psychiatry was to become my specialty, with barrio and ghetto slang my second language.

Quatro Flats was in a constant state of mild party. Any increase in activity quickly cranked up the intensity to serious party. At any hour of the day when the elevator doors opened on the fourth floor the soft aroma of marijuana would fill the elevator. This offended members of the administration who had some offices on this floor. The barrio brothers let the brass know they wanted their privacy. Quatro Flats was their home, to relax in as they pleased. I couldn't believe how they got away with it. Nursing administration ten years ago was made up mostly of women. I figure these women just didn't have the nerve to confront the men and tell them to shape up. Consequently, the men appeared to have a much higher failure rate than the women. Not all the men were constantly smoking pot and trying to get laid, I just don't remember any of the quiet studious ones (except for a few born agains, who would piously shake their heads as they walked through the halls).

Michael and I would hang out on the fourth floor about once a week. We were not considered regulars. Michael never smoked pot, and drank very little. The drink of the day was beer, lots of beer. I rank beer right there with lima beans and Brussels sprouts, totally disgusting. Gregory was frequently gallant and would pick up some wine for me. I think part of the reason Michael and I were not cool is that we were such party lightweights. This does not garner respect around a heavy duty crowd. A glass, or a glass and a half of wine is about my maximum; I smoked pot occasionally, but even this was not done in a serious enough manner to gain me any respect.

Partly I was being polite. I wasn't serious enough about pot to want to spend money buying it. I wasn't really clear what the social rules were around grass. I noticed people generally brought it with them and passed it around. If I didn't bring any, was it appropriate to smoke what was passed? If I smoked what was passed, wouldn't I eventually be expected to bring some? Where does one buy marijuana (definitely not at Bullocks)? If you can't buy it at Bullocks, you can't put it on a charge card, and this stuff is expensive. It got more complicated for me. If I didn't like the person who brought the pot, was I indebted to them if I smoked any? If I told people I didn't understand the rules, then they would know I was really out of it, and then I would feel stupid. I was stupid. I think most people knew I wasn't clear on how to proceed. They treated me like a sweet autistic child. They expected little of me, were delighted when I showed up, and knew I would leave early. I am always sleepy by ten p.m. Clearly I was not a party animal. I would like to really party and get wild, I just don't have the background or constitution for it.

Michael did not help my image at all. He drank even less than I did, unless he was morose. Then he did it in isolation, and to the point of oblivion. He was from a Jewish family and spent a period of his life as a born again Christian. The aura of a born again takes forever to wear off a person, even after they return to the real world. Michael still had a faint hint of zoned out saintliness hanging about him. It was only strong enough to put people off, but not strong enough for them to identify the source. Secretly, I would have liked to hang out with a really cool guy, who could add a degree of danger to my image. I tried loving the self-destructive sort once; this is truly hell on earth. I figure I am stuck with the image of wholesome and it's really what I do best.

Michael and I spent about nine months together lost in the joy of romance. Most of my first year of nursing school was spent in close connection with him. We went on day hikes, took two or three short trips together. We had a romantic week-end in San Francisco. I never grew accustomed to his politics, philosophy, or clothes. He always regarded me as something of an aberrant thinker. There is a limit to how long I can keep my eyes this tightly shut. My anxiety, frustrations, and fears grew, as I felt myself losing my delicate grasp on my closed lids.

Some people's eyelids fly open all at once with a start. Suddenly their vision is clear, and they are aghast at their situation. I tend to take the slower approach. Eventually the warm, pink mist in my head begins to clear. My vision starts to focus and the view is alarming. Sometimes I may try to squeeze my eyes back shut, but I have never found this to be effective. Mostly it is a feeling of loss. I will fight it as long as I can. The battle usually takes me several weeks before my eyes open to the point that I can no longer participate in the illusion. I have loved one or two so tenaciously the battle became a war that took my consciousness months to win. I guess I am lucky. I know people that need years to fully open their eyes and acknowledge what they see.

Chapter Sixteen

The Light of Day

It was an irritating dawn. Little by little, my patience grew thin. My soft gentle voice became grating, even to my ears. By the light of day, I looked around and realized my life was bereft of joy. I knew it wasn't Michael's fault. He was the same Michael he had always been. It was me, and the same old things that had bothered me about him all along. I suddenly felt like someone had thrown a bucket of cold water on my brain, washing away all traces of the rosy glow of romance. I was anguished. I was living with a horrible hang-over from a nine month, drunken binge on romance.

The end of romance is every lover's worst fear, and for good reason. Not only must one experience it, one must confess it to their lover. These are the worst times in my life. I had never experienced the death of someone I loved dearly. But the loss of romance had removed loved ones from my life at a frightening rate. One moment we were intimate, and the next we couldn't speak without heart-wrenching pain. I had experienced the loss enough times by now to know what I was in for. I was particularly sad with Michael, because he was such a good friend. The affection was not gone. The caring continued. I was a part of his life and he was a part of mine. It was only the romantic glow that was missing, the feeling of two hearts with wings, and the desire to make love.

I find sexual rushes are made of more delicate material than romantic feelings. The slender underpinnings of a sexual rush can be lost as quickly as an exhaled breath. Sometimes I can lose my sexual interest in a man before he even gets his shirt off. Each day with Michael I noticed more about him that bugged me. With each new irritation my desire to make love with him diminished. I wasn't eagerly waiting to hear his knock on my door; instead I felt trapped. I was waiting for a man to arrive who expected an entertaining evening with me topped off by some lively sex. I felt like a poodle who had grown tired of his hoop, jumping through it had become a chore.

My desire to make love had flown out the door on the heels of our romance. Since my inclination and skills for faking interest were not strong, Michael quickly assessed our relationship was changing. He put the question to me outright, "Do you want to stop seeing me?"

"No!" I cried, and I wasn't lying. "I want to see you, I just don't want to have sex with you anymore." Humpty Dumpty fell from the wall, our friendship lay in pieces all around us. I was emotionally on my knees scrambling for a way to piece it together again. Extricating sex and romance from a relationship without killing the friendship is almost impossible when the decision to do so is unilateral. I didn't want to lose my best friend at the same time I was losing my lover. Michael told me that was too bad because that was what I had just done.

Sex can be a very securing act. I wanted Michael in my life. If I took away the sex, how could I expect the rest? Men classically chill and run when a woman says, "I want to be dear friends with you, without sex," especially men with whom one has been sexual. My actions towards Michael became unclear and muddled. When I feared his loss, my anxiety rose, and suddenly I was having sexual feelings towards him. I would find myself touching his shoulder or leg, or sitting way too close to him. The confusion made us both crazy. I felt guilt and self-loathing. Michael expressed pain and anger.

There are a variety of ways of coping with romantic dissolution. I am a private person. I tend to downplay my romances so I can slide through the dissolution with as little public acclaim as possible. There are other styles. There is the blabber, who tells everyone who will listen every detail over and over. One of my worst fears is to go through a break-up with a blabber. I have broken up with a sobber. This was totally unexpected. Through our seven year relationship I never saw the man shed a tear. Once I broke up with him, he became Mr. Sensitivity. He left all his friends and work associates with soggy shoulder pads. The ways in which one can manage a public image at this time are endless. You can moan, sob, lie, or deny; you can pretend you don't care, you can pretend you never cared. The sobber went on to become religious. You can return home to mother. You can turn to Elizabeth Arden for a total make-over.

During our breakup I finally got an indication of the meaning behind Michael's style of dress. It was so obvious I can't believe I didn't see it all along. It was dramatic. A hat and floor length cape can only be described as dramatic. It isn't surprising I didn't pick up on this. Drama always strikes me as somewhat self-absorbed and pretentious. I sense a person is watching their life, rather than living it. I know this is an unfair label to plaster on the dramatic. The perfect approach for a man with a fondness for capes and hats who yearns for the return of chivalry and the round table, is to become morose. Mallory's Lancelot was Michael's hero. Michael did not wear his pain on his sleeve, he wore it on his chest as a breast plate. His sorrow was deeper and wider than Lancelot's. I never saw Michael's pain as artificial or trumped up, but it was horrifyingly public. He did the best Heathcliff I have ever seen. He reeked of gloom. He wore his agony around him like a cloak. It tore my heart to shreds to see him.

The most difficult aspect for me in breaking up is to have someone I love in pain and not be able to console them. Through all else in our relationship, Michael and I were able to hold each other in our pain. To be unable to reach out and take his head in my hands when he was hurt caused my heart to ache with anguish. Rarely can one deliver both the blow and the salve. Trying to do both intensifies the pain. For a while Michael and I did try to hold each other in our grief, but this became excruciating for us. We finally had to separate. We were each left to experience the loss of our romance individually.

I knew Michael better than any man I had known before, including my ex-husband. I knew many of his inner feelings, and some of his deepest fears. Total separation from him was very painful. I was left with observing him. Our proximity in the dorms ruled out privacy. Michael's flair for drama and flamboyance made him a hard act to avoid. If I were in a room with other people, you could count on Michael for morose entrances and flaming exits.

This intense and prolonged display of emotion did not garner Michael any respect from the other men on the fourth floor. People tire quickly of other people's agonies. This seems to be a fact few people in agony recognize. Michael's drama could be tolerated for a night or two, but several weeks was too much. When his mental morass lasted for several months, Michael was no longer considered a victim, but an asshole. I felt far too much guilt in this situation to show irritation or anger at him. I'm sure I must have felt both. He was behaving like a jerk and it was embarrassing for both of us.

Strangely, Michael's public displays of disdain for me caused others to feel quite warmly towards me. Gregory was protective. If Michael was going to act like a shit to me, then he wasn't welcome at the parties. This made socializing difficult for me. The main place to gather in the dorm was the fourth floor. Evelyn or Susan would invite me to join them for wine in Gregory's room. If Michael was there he would immediately storm out at my entrance. This would piss everyone off. I was angry at him for the childish behavior, but I also felt guilty that my presence was causing him greater isolation. I would go down to the fourth floor less often so Michael could socialize in peace. This caused people to have an increased irritation at him, and to seek me out more frequently.

After several months, Michael still continued to act out with displays of depression. Other people were becoming worried, and so was I. Susan spoke of going to see Dr. Stevens, the physician to the student nurses, about Michael. Stevens was a huge warm teddy bear of a man, and beloved by everyone and one of the best physicians I have ever known. Since I knew Michael the best, it seemed appropriate for me to go see Stevens. I told him of Michael's and my relationship, explained the break-up, and described Michael's current behavior. This had become a greater concern to many of us because we had just experienced another nursing student making a serious suicide attempt. She was now recovering in the critical care unit.

Information spreads fast in tight places. We knew about the suicide attempt. We all knew how the young woman had taken the signs and pictures off her dorm room door the day before her attempt. Dorm doors were used as billboards. We all expressed ourselves on our doors. Michael had taken to putting poems about death on his door. Most recently he had cleared his door off. It had been a very close call with the other woman. If she had been found an hour or two later, she wouldn't have lived. I shared with Dr. Stevens the messages Michael was putting out on his door.

I had a hard time making the decision whether to act on Michael's signals or not. I knew he would be extremely angry with me for involving a professional. However, I trusted Stevens' judgment far more than I did my own. Michael frightened me. I didn't know if his behavior was something I should take seriously or not. I did know that if I guessed wrong and did nothing, if Michael should kill himself, I would feel like a coward and would always regret my decision.

I was right about one thing Michael was angry with me beyond words. He felt violated. I had risked his career in nursing. How dare I? Saying "I dared to do this because I love you" doesn't cut it with an angry person. It took me a long time to become comfortable with my decision to involve Dr. Stevens. It wasn't until I worked on the adolescent crisis unit at County dealing with a great number of suicidal patients that I came to peace with the choice I made. If I were faced with a similar situation today my choice would be the same.

We only spoke occasionally after that. Our first year of nursing school had ended on a sad note. Twice, durring our second year, we were placed in the same clinic group. Michael transferred out both times. We met at the bulletin board at the beginning of a new semester. He noted that once again I had been placed in the best clinical group. It pissed him off; he couldn't understand it. He was the altruist with the humanitarian ethics. Why the hell was I the Cosmic Universe's favorite child? I don't know why. Sometimes, I think it's true. Sometimes, I feel guilty about it. All I could tell him was "I'm sorry."

Chapter Seventeen

"I Don't Know Nothin' 'Bout Birthin' No Babies"

We had now completed Nursing 101 and 102. We were halfway through our schooling at County. Our second year of nursing began with our class of one hundred being broken up into three groups, sections 201 A, B, and C. After these all that was left was Nursing 202 (Advanced Medical/Surgical) and graduation. For Nursing 201 our groups took turns rotating through pediatrics, obstetrics, and psychiatry. My first rotation was in obstetrics. Michael and I were in the same section, but with different clinical instructors. He showed up for that first day of class wearing a button, quoting Butterfly McQueen's famous line from **Gone With The Wind**. I loved his sense of humor, and his shared anxiety about birthin' babies. As the youngest daughter, and one of the younger cousins, it was true that I knew "nothin, 'bout birthin' no babies". My older sister Resa had two sons and we had spent hours on end together during her first pregnancy. This is when I learned of some of the horrors that can take place when a body is taken over by hormones and a fetus. I learned of hemorrhoids, the need to urinate every twenty minutes, and the sensation of feeling like an elephant that was never going to give birth. I was a true obstetrics innocent.

Most young girls get their early experiences of mothering playing house. As the youngest child the role of mother was not available to me. Resa always played Mother and she did a smashing job of it. From the beginning it was clear to all of us Resa would have no problem handling her children. Lucinda, my oldest sister, was a little different. Her preferred role was that of Father. This made sense to us. Being the oldest, she liked to be in charge. In our home this was definitely our Father's role; therefore she played Father. I had enough of playing baby, this was my normal family role. I chose to let one of my dolls play that part, while I took on the more challenging role of playing the family's trusted pet, Corky, "The Wonder Dog."

Playing Corky did give me some maternal experiences. Part of the Wonder of Corky was how well she took care of the baby when Mother was busy. This was a somewhat distorted picture of mothering, since I was mostly limited to carrying a doll around by it's nighty in my teeth. I didn't mind so much not getting to play Mother, because I loved the role of Corky. I played Corky, "The Wonder Dog" twenty-four hours a day, for four years. Kindergarten finally put an end to Corky, and we are all thankful. I think I instinctively knew that what my family would tolerate, the outside world would not.

Playing Corky did little to prepare me for Obstetrics. Mrs. Ramaswamy was the woman to guide me through my first encounters with the world of childbirth. We were again broken up into small clinical groups of about eight people. Mrs. Ramaswamy, a short, round faced, Indian woman was our clinical instructor. Her eyes and skin were dark in color which accentuated the whiteness of her smile. She wore her black hair in a small bun at the nape of her neck. Her normal dress was a sari, unless she was doing something that required a nurse's uniform. Mrs. Ramaswamy's nature was one of ultimate gentleness. She was a perfect teacher for learning the sensitive art of non-intrusive, supportive nursing care of a new baby and mother.

Lectures that semester were pretty much the routine Obstetrical/Gynecological stuff. I remember a couple of films on abortions and Cesarean births so graphic they caused me to leave the room. I got caught hanging out in the hall by the master instructor. She told me I ought to be watching the films. I told her they made me feel sick and queasy. She must have had a similar response to the films. She was too sympathetic to send me back.

Obstetrics was a truly fun rotation on the wards. I think most of us felt this way. We had seen so much pain, trauma, loss, and death on our other rotations that this was a picnic. I felt like a fortunate guest, invited into these women's lives, momentarily, to share in their joy. My first three weeks in OB were spent in the pre-partum unit. This was for women who were having difficult pregnancies, or were expecting difficult births.

Many of the women on this unit were diabetic and their pregnancies required close monitoring. This is where I learned to use a doppler to amplify the sounds heard through the stethoscope. I would fumble around with the machinery trying to figure out how to use it, while my patient would give me advice. I enjoyed this teamwork. Many of the women were new at having babies, I was new at nursing pregnant women. We experimented and learned together. I would work with a mother to try and hear her baby's heartbeat. I would mess with the machine, she would show me the best place to listen. When we would finally hear that rapid little beat, we would both laugh with excitement.

We would talk about her expectations. If this were her first child, I would share with her my still limited knowledge on the process of birth. I would listen to her questions and return the next day with answers I had looked up. If she was a mother with lots of experience, she would enlighten me on the realities of childbirth. The pre-partum floor at County hums with excitement and expectation. Ten years ago, County was one of the best places in the state for handling a complicated pregnancy.

During this part of my rotation we also spent time at satellite clinics serving the community with prenatal care. I was assigned for a day to follow a mid-wife on her rounds seeing patients. The mid-wives were nurses with additional education in obstetrics and gynecology. They worked at the clinics and were assigned women who's pregnancies showed no signs of complication. The mid-wife was responsible for a woman's prenatal treatment, delivery, and postpartum care. The woman I was assigned to follow was small, with frizzy red hair, and a New York Bronx accent. She was bright, well educated, hyper, and harried. Her name was Sue, and she welcomed me warmly.

I was impressed with Sue, impressed with her air of competence. Her confidence seemed to go bone deep. The birthing of babies was a mystery to me. I understood the vague principle that everything down there opens up and the baby comes out. I also knew there was pain and blood, and the terrible possibility of lethal complications. Later, in my chiropractic studies, I began to understand the natural order of the process. I saw the beauty of the body, working in synchronized rhythm with itself and the baby, requiring no assistance from the outside. This doesn't mean I would care to go through the process of giving birth alone, but the thought no longer terrifies me. I can see the symmetry and the order now.

Ten years ago the medical community still regarded pregnancy as a form of disease, a state of being requiring intervention by trained professionals, high-tech equipment, medication, and hospitalization. The mid-wives were the forerunners of a return to sense and sensibility. Sue didn't stand away from her patients and speak in medical jargon. She spoke to the women in simple straightforward language. She explained what was going on, described their options, allowed women to make their own choices. She supported and assisted her patients in the choices they made.

I had observed Sue with two patients. Just before we were to enter the third examining room she stopped me. She told me the next case was going to be interesting. The woman spoke no English, was not married or employed, and Sue now had to tell her she is expecting twins. I cringed and felt weak, frightened and guilty all at once. The unfairness of life, the cruelty of fate, and the easiness of my own life in comparison left me feeling like a ghoulish observer of another's misfortune. I walked in the door like a dog with my tail between my legs, an apology on my lips.

Sue walked in confidently, ready to deal with the business at hand. This wasn't a catastrophe, this was life, and life is sometimes hard. She spoke in Spanish, explaining to the woman that the results of the ultrasound test showed "dos bambinos". "Dos bambinos?" "Si, dos bambinos."

Sue remained quiet for a few moments to let the woman collect her thoughts. Anxiety and concern crossed the young woman's face, while Sue remained solid and available. Nobody panicked, nobody cried.

My anxiety over the situation cleared enough for me to look around and notice a young girl about five sitting in the corner. Sue spoke to the little girl and explained that her mother was going to have two babies. Her mother would need her help and support around the house. The little girl looked solemn, and nodded her head that she understood. She then moved her chair over closer to her mother. Sue explored with the mother any possibility of support from the father. The young woman shook her head firmly and said "no help". Sue rose and took her patient's hand. She spoke in Spanish so I only picked up a little of what was said. This would be harder, but the woman must begin making plans. The front desk would give her the names and addresses of agencies that might be of help.

I followed Sue through her rounds for the rest of the day. I was exhausted at the end of eight hours. I had gained tremendous respect for County's outpatient Ob/Gyn clinics. I felt the patients were fortunate to have the quality of care provided by the mid-wives. I realized I was a long way away from wanting to take on the responsibility assumed by the mid-wives. I also felt incredibly light and unencumbered. I didn't have Sue's job, I didn't have a five year old child, I wasn't expecting twins, my life seemed like a breeze. I felt a small stab of guilt, but mostly relief as I drove back to the hospital.

Birthing babies came next. I was scared. Other than baby chickens pecking their way out of eggs, I had never seen any births, no kittens, puppies or guppies. T.V. and the movies were my only exposure to this process. Hollywood does not make giving birth look very appealing. I mostly recalled women screaming and heaving in agony, clutching at other people, babies and women dying in childbirth, or tears of joy, as a baby cries somewhere in the background.

The first birth I was able to observe was a Cesarean section, more commonly called a C-section. This was sort of a double whammy for me, birth and surgery all at once. It was on the spur of the moment, Mrs. Ramaswamy grabbed me and several others, saying, "quick, over here." I never liked it when this happened. When nursing instructors get all fired up, and want you to hurry up and follow them, they are usually leading you to observe some infrequent, very messy, often disgusting procedure. We were rushed into a tiny room the size of a linen closet. The wall on the right had a large glass window and a couch pushed up against it. Seven of us were crammed into this room, while a small, excited Mrs. Ramaswamy told us how lucky we were.

She instructed us to climb up on the sofa and look in the window. We had been given permission to observe a C-section. Our timing was perfect, they were just about to make the incision. Beyond being pregnant, the woman was also obese. Surgery on the obese is not a pretty sight. Having the opportunity of watching someone's abdomen cut open is not my idea of great luck. Being served chocolate pudding in the cafeteria is a lucky thing. This surgery was gross, and I was beginning to feel sick. It looked like this was going to take a while, so I stepped down and asked someone to tell me when they got to the baby. I didn't want to miss my first birth.

Mrs. Ramaswamy looked disappointed in me when she saw me sitting on the couch at my comrades' feet, trying to control the sweats. I told her I would get up as soon as it was time for the baby to come out. "OK, quick, it's coming, here it is!" I jumped up, elbowed my way in, in time to see it. Bloody, squirming, and crying, it was a baby. I took a couple of breaths and enjoyed the miracle of birth via surgery. The baby was handed off to a nurse and the doctor returned to deal with the mother.

I had thought it was safe to come up on the couch I had thought the worst was over. I had no idea that after the baby was delivered the doctor would take the woman's uterus out of her abdominal cavity, and place it on her stomach to check it out. Mrs. Ramaswamy explained that he was looking for any tears that might need repair. That did it. I had over-identified with the patient. The thought of my uterus, sitting on my stomach while someone examined it, completely undid me. My head started to swim. The room got bright, then dark. I was covered in sweat. I had sunk from my observation point on the couch, to sitting with my head between my knees. Mrs. Ramaswamy was not impressed, but she did let me forego the next lucky opportunity to observe a C-section.

During the labor and delivery section of obstetrics, you never knew if you would be lucky enough to see a birth. You were assigned to one of three rooms: labor, delivery, or postpartum. If your patient in labor advanced to the delivery room you got to go with her and watch the birth. I started in the labor room. My first patient was not very far along in her labor. An intern came in and prepared to put a fetal monitor on the baby. This did not look like a pleasant experience for the baby or the mother. The monitor would record the infant's heart rate up to the moment of delivery.

The intern held a long tube with a wire running through it that was connected to a monitor. There was a small screw on the other end of the wire. The tube is run up the mother's vagina, to the dilated cervix, where hopefully the baby's head is presenting. You also hope it's the top of the baby's head and not its little face, because this is where the doctor is going to screw in the wire. Baby's first welcome to the world, a screw in it's head. Now the mother must lie in bed on her back through the rest of her labor, because she is hooked up to a monitor.

We were given a cursory description of how to read the monitor and what symptoms to observe for in the mother. There were real nurses around, supervising and checking on everything. But frequently I was left alone with my patient for what seemed like an eternity, about fifteen to twenty minutes. The whole point of the hospital is to be there in case something goes wrong. Other than that, the process of giving birth goes on whether you want it to or not. I was to be on guard for signs of complications. I felt the best I could do was to try not to be a complication. So I politely declined when the gracious intern offered me the exciting opportunity of screwing the monitor wire into the baby's head. "Dear God," I thought, "should I ever become pregnant, please don't let some idiot student nurse screw a wire into my baby's head."

Towards the end of my first day in the labor room, Mrs. Ramaswamy rushed up to me, grabbed my arm, and told me to follow her. I reluctantly joined the train of white ducks, following her to observe another gruesome sight. We were taken to an area with a couple of sinks and told to scrub up. Scrub up! I was so excited, just like in the movies. We were already wearing surgical clothing. Everyone working labor and delivery changed into surgical scrubs and plastic shoe covers before entering the unit. I liked this. I liked the cut of the surgical scrub dresses. The ones small enough to fit me were always pretty short, and I thought my legs looked attractive. Never one to let a fashion moment go by, I had carefully explored all two of the surgical scrub options, and found the style most flattering to me.

In the days of Dr. Kildare and Ben Casey, doctors and nurses wore those tight fitting cloth caps on their heads. These caps had dignity. The outfit was completed with a cloth mask tied at the top and bottom, and on the women, plenty of eye make-up. My suite mate Susan had already been in a surgical theater. She told me that the nurses wore lots of eye make-up, and always had beautiful eyes. She guessed it might be a prerequisite for being a surgical nurse or a woman surgeon. I assured myself I was not in nursing school to lure a male doctor's attention away from his patient on the table. But I was not going to miss an opportunity to look as smashing as possible in an outfit I had admired on T.V. for years. The fantasy of Richard Chamberlin, looking up and becoming transfixed by my beautiful, compassionate eyes, was too good to miss. My eye make-up was impeccable every day of labor and delivery.

So finally, here we were, told to scrub up. I was really excited. Everyone was talking about seeing a birth. I couldn't wait to see how I looked in this outfit. I headed straight for the special cap and mask. The shelves were loaded with these ugly, green, paper shower caps. The masks were a conical shape, made of white filter paper, and they were secured by an elastic band. I figured the good stuff had to be around here somewhere. I was determined to find it. Everyone around me was grabbing and putting on this ugly stuff. I kept searching. Finally, someone asked, "What are you looking for?" I was embarrassed to tell them. I vaguely said, "I thought there might be some other caps." "Nope, that's it, better hurry."

With that, another beloved fantasy was blown. I had missed the days of beautiful, dignified, surgical clothes. By the time I had put on the transparent plastic booties, green shower cap, white paper mask, and surgical gloves, I looked as horrible as everybody else, and was now late. My mind was eager to avoid all comparison to those old T.V. fantasy pictures. This left me free to focus on the business at hand, the birthing of a baby.

I squeezed my way into an already packed delivery room. The focus of everyone's attention was the delivery table in the center of the room. The mother to be was lying on her back, her legs strapped into those cold metal stirrups beloved by all women. The number of people in the room surprised me. I must have been one of fifteen others there to observe this woman giving birth. This is the price one pays for medical care at a county teaching facility, the loss of privacy. I was later to observe other deliveries that were much more private. But my first experience in the delivery room was pretty much a circus.

Though the mother had no privacy, with everyone trying to get a good look, the event was still a miracle. The room was not a quiet place filled with decorum. People were excited. As the baby's head crowned and began to push forward the excitement grew. Jaded, over-educated doctors and nurses began shouting "It's coming, the baby's coming." "Here's the baby, it's a boy. You've got a boy Mrs. Garcia." We all shoved and pushed each other to get a first glimpse of the baby. Blood and guts make me sick, but newborn babies, even bloody and dripping look just wonderful. Their smashed little faces, crying indignantly, hold the excitement of a brand new fresh life.

I was given the job of weighing the baby. At that time babies were not given immediately to their mothers to begin nursing if they chose. Baby's first interaction was with the staff. I was the person to weigh him, at eight pounds he was a big plump boy. He was then wrapped in a blue blanket. Babies were immediately color coded, his genitalia at birth to determine his color preferences for life. The State of California required a final insult to it's newest resident before being handed over to his mother. By law the baby's eyes had to receive drops of silver nitrate. This was to prevent the baby from being blinded in case it had come into contact with syphilis during its passage through it's mother's vagina.

This is a controversial procedure. Many doctors, including Robert S. Mendelsohn, M.D., author of **Male Practice,** felt silver nitrate was not only barbaric, but unnecessary. A blood test will tell you if the mother has syphilis, so I never could see the necessity of insulting all babies in this manner.

After about ten minutes this baby had been footprinted, weighed, wrapped up, and temporarily blinded he could now be lovingly turned over to his mother. Once we laid this small boy in the arms of his mother we became outsiders. Their connection to each other was so intimate and intense, that we became superfluous. Mother and baby looked like they had known each other a long time. For ten minutes this baby had belonged to all of us. In my moment alone with him at the scales I was one of the first people to talk to him, and tell him about the world. I only told him that the scale was cold, and that he was beautiful. I told him he weighed eight pounds, and that I was glad to see him. That was all the time I had. I felt involved with his life, until I saw him in his mother's arms, and realized my part was less than insignificant.

I have since wondered what other people secretly whisper to babies. Is it the mysteries of life poured into their ears, or merely nonsense and gibberish? I believe babies, dogs, cats, and horses are good for the soul. They give me an ear into which I can whisper secrets.

I was lucky during my rotation on labor and delivery, I was able to see six or seven births. Most of these births were last minute rushes into the delivery room, much like my first experience. Maria Hernandez was the only patient I was able to follow from labor to delivery. I was excited when I was assigned Maria because she was well along in her labor, so she would probably deliver during my shift. I walked in and introduced myself to my patient.

Maria was twenty-two years old and expecting her second child. I quickly noticed that a woman who is two hours away from delivering a baby, and currently in intense labor pains, is not very interested in meeting a new face. Maria spoke no English. During a break in the pains she smiled at me for a moment, and reached for my hand. This touched my heart completely. I felt immediately connected to this woman. We were two women having an international coffee moment. I felt she would always remember me as the gentle nurse who held her hand through her labor pains.

At this time most of the women delivering at County had no prenatal care, no Lamaze classes, no education on childbirth. You just waited until the pains got real bad, walked into County, and had a baby. Alternative birthing rooms were just being explored with the mid-wives. These patients could have their families with them. But most of our patients were alone through their labor and delivery. I felt all warm and misty holding Maria's hand during her time of stress, separated from family and friends.

The special glow of our connection lasted about one and a half minutes, until the next spasm of labor gripped Maria's gut. Then her hand clamped down on mine like a vice and she squeezed, and squeezed, and squeezed. The woman was strong, and insensible to my anguish. I panicked and began to scream with her, "Ahhh," we both yelled together. Finally the labor pain passed and Maria released her death grip.

People react differently to pain, some are stoic, others are babies. There is the type that goes white and silent. I tend to use the focus-off method. I acknowledge the pain, then try to distract my mind and focus elsewhere. If it gets really bad I may even become a joker. This is the sad case of the person cracking jokes to avoid crying or panic. Maria's tools for dealing with pain were screaming histrionics. I had just enough time to calm myself, speak a few soothing words to Maria, as a way of focusing off my pain, before the next wave of contractions hit.

I quickly removed my hand from hers, and held onto the side of her bed. I tried to speak reassuringly to her, which is tough when all I had available was my broken Spanish. Maria never heard me or saw me. She screamed and grabbed for my hand. God, she was fast; if I didn't give her my hand she would go for my arm. "Ahhhhh," we both started yelling together again. Then I remembered what I had been told by an intern in the cafeteria. At the time, I had thought he was being a sexist creep, so I ignored him. Now, I was searching my brain for his infinite wisdom. He had said women in labor would squeeze your hand and break it if you didn't watch out. He said the trick was to give them one finger, because no matter how hard they squeezed, they couldn't damage one outstretched finger.

I abandoned my dislike for this intern. I pried open Maria's hand, released my now crippled one, and inserted one index finger. I accomplished this maneuver during a break in the spasms. At the next wave of pain Maria gripped my finger. She found that rather unsatisfying and tried to get a hold on more of my fingers, but I out-maneuvered her. Another nurse, possibly a smarter nurse, would have backed the hell away from Maria, and stayed out of arm's reach. I couldn't do it, I didn't have the heart. I couldn't leave Maria with no hand to hold. So for two hours we did a dance. The pain would come and Maria's hands would gobble at mine looking for something to crush. I kept inserting one outstretched finger as a donation into her eager fist.

Finally we got the word Maria was far enough along we could wheel her into the delivery room. An intern and I scrubbed up while Maria was strapped to the table. It was a hectic day at the hospital and I noticed there wasn't going to be the usual crowd of students around to watch this birth. Once I got into the delivery room I realized it was busier than I had thought. There was an intern assigned to this room and an R.N. who was an old hand at delivering babies, but she was required to assist in two adjoining rooms at once. Despite all Maria's noise her delivery was routine and uncomplicated, so the intern and I were left to do this alone.

The intern and I said hello and assumed our positions. I was at Maria's head, he was between her legs. So far so good. We then both simultaneously experienced that moment when the brain goes dead, and you have no idea what the hell to do next. I know this event was simultaneous because he looked up at me just as I looked up at him, and two frozen, blank stares met one another. Maria saved us; she let out a blood curdling yell that threw us both into action.

Maria's baby was strong and healthy. She was determined to come into the world, regardless of the fact that she had two nincompoops here to assist her. Maria yelled and screamed as her daughter pushed her way into the light. All that was required of the intern was that he hold out his hands and catch the baby. He managed to do this flawlessly. Upon the arrival of the baby, the trained R.N. magically appeared. She scooped up the baby, took care of the formalities, and filled out the paperwork, placed the baby in Maria's arms, and disappeared before the intern and I had quite figured out that the baby was here and fine.

Maria held her baby close to her chest, but showed no inclination to nurse her. I have heard women friends tell me they had gone numb to the pain by the time the baby was delivered. This was not the case for Maria. She continued to scream in agony. The piercing yells every few seconds were beginning to make me crazy. I told the intern ,"This woman needs some Demerol". He responded with "Yeah, I'll get her some, but I'm busy right now." He was busy delivering the placenta, and then moving on to repairing the episiotomy, a surgical incision to widen the opening for the baby's head to come out.

The intern kept working, Maria kept screaming, and I was the one who finally couldn't take it any more. Doctors are the only ones allowed to order medications. I didn't care. I'd had it. I used my most authoritative voice and yelled over Maria's cries, "This woman deserves some Demerol, now!" A really good authoritative voice brings out the obedient child in most of us. The intern had been well trained to respond. Within moments Maria had fifty cc's of medication on board. We were all praying for peace. Without classes or preparation, Maria had just gone through natural childbirth. She didn't appear to be enjoying it one bit. As the meds went in, between shouts, she said "gracias."

The rest was routine. Our patient quieted down enough to take a good long look at her baby. With the pain subsiding Maria was beginning to show signs of delight in her newborn. The intern finished up his stitching. Maria was stable and ready to be wheeled into the postpartum room for observation. My shift was ending. My last view of Maria was of her being wheeled out of the room, a little groggy, smiling and holding her new daughter.

The last few weeks of my obstetrics rotation were spent on the postpartum floor. Women's hospital at County was newer and set up with semi-private rooms. The first week I was assigned one mother and one baby. Later our load was increased to two mothers and their babies. This was a fun time to be involved in obstetrics, because it was a time of the resurgence of common sense. Natural birth had been in vogue in private hospitals for a while but it was just now beginning to trickle down to the masses at the county level.

Breast-feeding was experiencing a renaissance. Doctors were not aware of this yet, but nurses were onto it and hot. It was the perfect solution to meet many of our patients' needs. Free, portable baby food that doesn't require sterilization, refrigeration, or heating up; what a great idea! Interestingly, this great idea had been out of use for so long that people had forgotten how to do it. Over- read yuppie mothers, who had studied every child care book ever written rarely need more education on breast-feeding. They could write essays on it. But our patients were busy with paying the rent, and doing what needed to be done to survive. They were not up to date on the latest in child care technologies, like breast-feeding.

Many of our patients thought breast-feeding was backwards and primitive. There was a myriad of myths and confusion surrounding this practice that had to be sorted out. Many nurses deeply believe that a primary part of their job is the role of patient educator and advocate. This is an area where many R.N.'s would like to spend a lot more time if they weren't so overloaded already. As students, we had the luxury of a small workload, so we could practice nursing as it was intended. I believe the loss of this one-on-one time to work with patients in a quality manner has been the cause of much of the dissatisfaction in the profession today. As students we did not know how much we would miss the opportunity to provide truly high quality care to our patients once we hit the "real world". Administrators have never figured out that this is what makes a nurse feel fulfilled in work.

Our instructors encouraged us to move quickly. We had to educate our patients on breast-feeding as soon as the baby was born. This was because we only had a window of forty-eight to seventy-two hours before a well meaning intern, following his superior's instructions, offered to inject the new mother with medication to dry up her milk production. An M.D.'s education often lags a few years behind nursing education on the psychosocial issues. Nurses are usually generous people, more than willing to share their wealth of information with doctors. After sharing their information with doctors repeatedly and insistently for a long enough time, doctors will generally hear what nurses are saying.

My first new mother on the postpartum unit was a young Mexican woman, Connie, who spoke no English. She was a beautiful girl with lovely eyes, smiling like a Madonna as she held her new baby. I spent the morning taking care of Connie. We used gestures to talk to one another. Together we admired and played with her new son. By ten o'clock Mrs. Ramaswamy wanted to know if I had educated my patient on breast-feeding yet. I hadn't. I didn't know much about breast-feeding and what I did know I couldn't translate. I felt awkward telling another woman what she should do with her breast. Besides, I wasn't really sure what she should do other than stick it in the baby's mouth, and I hadn't learned how to say that.

Mrs. Ramaswamy was alarmed. This woman delivered two days ago. The interns would be offering her a shot to dry up her milk any minute, we must hurry. I felt kind of ridiculous rushing off as the good fairy of breast milk when I really didn't know much about the whole thing. Mrs. Ramaswamy saw my hesitation and took my arm. She gave me a warm smile, and said she would come with me and help. She was wearing her sari that day. She looked like a loving, gentle earth mother from the East. I was tremendously thankful for her presence.

We entered Connie's room where she was sitting up in bed playing with her son. I introduced her to Mrs. Ramaswamy, who spoke English in a soft Indian accent. Connie smiled without understanding a word. I sympathized, sometimes I had trouble understanding Mrs. Ramaswamy's English too. Mrs. Ramaswamy began explaining about breast-feeding in broken English to a woman who spoke no English. I would attempt to translate this into my own version of broken Spanish. My instructor held Connie's son in one hand and her own full breast in the other as demonstration. I lamely repeated these gestures on my breast. Connie watched, intrigued with our display, but comprehending none of it.

Mrs. Ramaswamy was determined and we were all beginning to warm up to our confusing subject. The baby was handed to me, while Mrs. Ramaswamy began to open the front of Connie's gown, to expose her left breast. I was instructed to place the baby at Connie's breast. Embarrassed and awkward, I sat on the bed next to Connie and attempted to place the baby's mouth on her breast. Connie laughed, she understood, but shook her head to let us know she didn't have any idea of what she should do. Mrs. Ramaswamy was excited, we had made contact. She climbed up on the bed on the other side of Connie so she could get her hands into the action.

Now we three had a shared goal, we wanted the baby to drink. We laughed and prodded Connie's son. Mrs. Ramaswamy tickled his cheek to stimulate sucking. It seemed like a good idea, so Connie and I joined in. In three languages we encouraged and teased him. "Come on baby, drink baby." This much determination was too much to resist. Connie's son began to suck. His action surprised her; Connie was laughing in shock and delight. Mrs. Ramaswamy and I were excited, we were laughing and encouraging him. If he stopped for a moment we all went back to tickling and cooing and proffering Connie's breast in an enticing manner.

Luckily hospital beds are strong, and able to accommodate three laughing women and a baby. Connie's son delighted the three of us by nursing for ten minutes before he fell asleep. We sat quietly for a while and watched him, before Mrs. Ramaswamy and I finally climbed off the bed and gave Connie some peace. I don't know if Connie decided to continue nursing, or if an intern came in the next day and gave her a shot. However, I remember our day together clearly; it was one of my most memorable experiences in obstetrics.

Our six weeks in obstetrics came to an end. I had thoroughly enjoyed the rotation. It is compulsory that when any rotation ends students must party. These were not raucous blowouts on Quatro Flats. This would be a more civilized lunch out with our instructors. It was late Spring and we were going to an outdoor restaurant that had a patio and garden area capable of seating a hundred or so. This was a Mexican restaurant complete with a strolling mariachi band. Mrs. Ramaswamy had a tradition of dressing the women in her group in saris for their final celebration.

Our turn had come. We were ready to don our saris and drink Margaritas. We finished our work on the wards early that day at noon. We immediately met in the dorms to get dressed in our outfits. Mrs. Ramaswamy had brought two armloads of beautiful fabrics, with exotic prints and colors. She had told us to wear short sleeved T-shirts in solid colors. We stood around in our underwear and T-shirts discussing, debating, and conniving who would get to wear what. I had worn an orange T-shirt and had managed, without defacing anyone, to find a fabric with orange and emerald green that looked nice with my shirt.

Mrs. Ramaswamy went around and wrapped each woman in her sari. The method of wrapping had everything to do with whether or not your clothing stayed on. It happened too fast for me to figure out how she did it. She wrapped the fabric tightly around my hips, there was a twist and a fold creating a drape across my chest, and leaving fall of surplus fabric behind my left shoulder. There were nine of us all dressed up in costume. We looked like we were going to a theme party. A sari is a compelling form of dress on an Indian woman, with her dark eyes, hair, and skin setting off a gleaming white smile. Even Mrs. Ramaswamy's small round figure had dignity and grace in her sari. We were a group of blondes and brunettes, not an exotic beauty in the bunch. We looked like a gang of overage, waspish Girl Scouts, out to earn a merit badge in Eastern Lore.

But there is courage and communion in numbers. The nine of us lied and told each other how great we looked. This way we could rely on the security of our gang to take our fully costumed act out for public display. The lies were a necessary aid until the margaritas took over and numbed us to our true appearance.

The garden of the restaurant was packed with about seventy members of our class. People table hopped and compared their rotations while munching down burritos and enchiladas. I finished up my obstetrics rotation wearing a sari and eating guacamole dip. We raised our glasses in a toast, "Farewell and thank you Mrs. Ramaswamy. And now, on to pediatrics."

Chapter Eighteen

A Play Siren Searches For A Pal

There were many gaps in my life created by the loss of Michael. I was now out a lover, a best friend, and most of all, someone to answer my siren's call of, "come play with me". Evelyn is pretty good at answering my call to play, especially if the call is for shopping and lunch, preferably in Beverly Hills. But I have a lot of play needs. I had to get realistic about who was most likely to give in to which tantalizing call, and then give them my very best shot. I have been told this is my greatest talent, calling loved ones away from things they should be doing.

Personally I am not sure if this is one of my best traits or one of my worst. My friends tell me I'm bad, complain occasionally about my lack of a work ethic, but frequently answer the call and come play with me. Our lives change and our responsibilities to the outside world shift. Some of my loved ones have become unavailable for spontaneous play. I am fortunate; so far my life continues to evolve in ways that allow me more freedom, not less. It seems like that is the appropriate reward for growing up, to become more free. As I watch my friends, I realize this is not the case for most people. I am looking forward to about fifteen years from now. If I am lucky, there will be enough play left in them that they'll take early retirements; then I can seduce my friends all over again.

While in nursing school I knew who I could put the touch on to meet my various play needs. Evelyn understands the need to purchase an item of clothing that is frivolous, impractical, almost totally unusable, and looks absolutely smashing. She can be trusted never to encourage me in pursuing something that is unflattering. Her eye is critical in the areas that count. How does it make my ass look? Do my breasts look great? And best of all, something has to go right up to the edge of scandal before Evelyn would speak the words "too short, too low cut, too bright, or too tight." I love Evelyn because she has never even pretended to guess how much wear I would get out of a particular item.

Susan was able to fill in some of the gaps left by Michael's absence. She wasn't into movies or dining out, and she rarely shopped. But she liked to watch movies on T.V. while eating Minestrone soup with bread and cheese. I wasn't a big fan of this type of soup, but I'll take movies under almost any condition. I even ate lentil soup while watching "Little House on the Prairie". That was the bottom limit for me. The two combined barely totaled up enough fun points to merit the taste of the soup.

The reason I frequently accepted Susan's generous offer of soup and bread was because I liked her companionship. The closeness and camaraderie of sitting on her twin bed together, sharing canned soup and bad T.V., made me feel cared for. I was hungry enough for this feeling that I have probably sat through ten hours of "Little House on the Prairie." I almost began to care if little blind Mary would ever see again or not.

With extra time on my hands I began to look around at the other faces in our nursing class for potential play partners. One man's face consistently showed up smiling and it belonged to Sam. He was the cutest man in our class. I know that 'cute man' is almost an oxymoron; boys, bunny rabbits, and babies are cute. Men and women hopefully are more profound. But cute fits Sam. He had tremendous sweetness and charm, and a wonderful sense of personal aesthetics. Sam looks like a young Geraldo Rivera suffused with warmth and a loving nature, if you can possibly imagine such a thing. As I look at his picture now, the sweetness and vulnerability are there in his face. Everybody liked Sam. Nobody really knew him, but everyone liked him.

Sam was not only cute and sweet, but he was cool. He had a lean body and a nice ass. His shirts were white and starched, with the long sleeves rolled up; or close fitting polo shirts (only the real ones by Ralph). His jeans were skin tight and always perfectly worn in to a fine, pale blue patina in the crotch. Fortunately, the picture I have of him is three-quarter length, so I get the full effect. His ties were very narrow, frequently leather. His hair was perfectly cut to follow the curve of his thick black waves. Part of his coolness came from appearing inaccessible. Though he lived on the fourth floor with the rest of the men he was rarely around. We would just catch glimpses of Sam taking off for unknown parts in a great looking outfit and wonder where he was going.

Somewhere during the course of Obstetrics, Sam and I had become friends. We were in the same clinical group. One day we finished our morning work at the same time and decided to have lunch together. As friends we fit together like a hand and glove. An accidental lunch quickly turned into planning our lunch times together. He got my jokes, he went to movies, he ate out, and he certainly knew where to shop. The perfect play team was born.

I did start to develop a bit of a crush on Sam, but one wonders about a man with such great taste. Apparently, no one wondered about this but me; everyone else seemed to know. We went to the movies one night and Sam talked about having children. He was from a Catholic family and knew his mother was waiting for grandchildren. It doesn't matter what kind of family you are from, I think everybody I knew had parents waiting for grandchildren. We talked about the pros and cons, the desire to please those we love, the desire to remain unburdened, same old stuff. The whole time I was running a monologue in my head, is this man gay or straight?

Sam and I intently discussed possibilities of parenting, while I silently debated his sexual preferences. I don't know why I didn't just ask him. I've never had qualms about asking other people. But Sam was so sweet I didn't want to be rude. I didn't want to hear what I probably already knew. Which, in retrospect, would have been some of the best news I could have gotten. Here was a relationship I couldn't goof up by taking it to romantic places when we were meant to be friends. I don't think I even really wanted to go to bed with Sam, I was just wondering if we eventually would. I have probably screwed up a lot of relationships just wondering such stupid stuff.

About a week after our first movie date my hair started driving me nuts. Some people have anxiety attacks that occur unpredictably at any moment; I have hair attacks. Suddenly, at eight o'clock at night I had to do something about my hair. A hair attack requires immediate intervention; something must be done to profoundly change my hair. Immediacy is important because if I put it off the need will abate, and I will miss the wonderful fulfillment of instant gratification. I instinctively know I must act quickly. This is how I know I am having a hair attack, as opposed to experiencing the angst of every day unruly hair. I have chosen desperate options at these times. I have talked my way into exclusive hair salons, "This is an emergency, I must be seen today", and then paid tremendous amounts of money to have strange things done to my hair. I have gone to unknown hairdressers at the bottom of the line department stores. I have paid people to perform previously untried techniques on my hair. More than once I have hit the home perm row at Save-On's.

Hair attacks can be tremendously satisfying in the moment, but living with the results is often protracted and painful. Short hair encourages such action because I rationalize, "it will grow out in a few months." I know that hair attacks are simply manifestations of my deep-seated self-dissatisfaction. However, knowing this does not make hair attacks go away.

Eight o'clock at night in the barrio is a tough time to get a hair attack. The salons on Rodeo are closed, and anyway to get there would be life-threatening. The local salons only do corn rows, and as Evelyn had pointed out, my hair hasn't the body to sustain this look. I thought of Sam. Sam was the only person at County that I knew who liked to draw and paint. I also draw and paint. I figured if you can be artistic in one area, you can be artistic in another. My hair attack was mostly focused on the back of my hair, too long, so I couldn't cut it myself without serious risk. I grabbed my scissors and went downstairs to bang on Sam's door.

I explained my theory to him, that being able to do one thing means you can probably do another. I told him he had innate talent - look how well he dresses. Sam was skeptical. It didn't sound like a good idea to him. I might not like the cut. I tried to explain that liking the cut was not as important as the experience of getting it cut. I did better when I returned to focusing on his innate talent. I can be persuasive when necessary. Sam gave in, and began to cut my hair.

Ten minutes into the job the phone rang. Sam's best friend Ronnie was calling to chat. Ronnie was a hair dresser, and he totally panicked when he heard what we were doing. Sam placated his friend quickly and got back to work. I was right, he was able to make the jump from working with the two dimensional to the three dimensional just fine. We were doing great, cruising along. I had a mirror and was giving advice and encouragement. Ronnie couldn't let go of what was happening in his absence. He called Sam again and offered to cut my hair for free, if I would just wait until tomorrow. Sam's tone was too reassuring, too soft, too warm, for this to be a buddy. I got the feeling that Ronnie's panic was not professional concern for my hair, but personal worry over what I might be doing with Sam. By the third phone call, my hair cut was finished. I looked good, and I no longer wondered about Sam's sexual preferences.

Sam was a West Side boy, I am an East Side girl. County is in the middle. County looms massive and spread out, slightly to the east of central downtown L.A. Nobody in L.A. is a downtown type of person, if they can help it. We would all rather get in our cars and drive for hours to be an East Side or a West Side, or God forbid, a Valley kind of person. Each area claims to be the only civilized area in L.A. County to live.

A true East Sider, West Sider, or Valleyite, does not live in these areas for economic reasons, available housing, or accessibility. It appears to be more of a philosophical, social, and aesthetic statement on how life is lived. This is an account given by an East Side woman. I won't talk about the Valley much, because we East Siders agree with the West Siders on one issue: the Valley exists as a crowded corridor between the East and the West, having no intrinsic value of its own. This is a harsh view, I know. It is also a bonding point between the East and the West. It is also this view that makes the Valleyites think the rest of us are tremendous snobs. Which is, of course, the whole point after all. It is perfectly appropriate to be snobbish about being self-actualized enough to realize the East Side is the only place for true quality of life in L.A.

Pasadena, South Pasadena, Arcadia, San Marino, and Sierra Madre are the cities that epitomize the East Side. Traditionally one thinks of conservative, old, white money when they hear these names. San Marino has the most prominent John Birch Society I have ever seen. The cars are Volvos and Mercedes station wagons, big safe things. The feeling is small town. The streets are heavily lined with jacarandas, magnolias, eucalyptus, and liquid amber trees. The sidewalks are raised and treacherous from all the roots. The homes are older, many fifty to a hundred years old, which is about as old as they get in L.A. There are big front lawns, with huge shade trees, and children's toys are scattered everywhere.

Pasadena is old, with a sense of tradition, permanence and taste. No gaudy Christmas decorations here. Seasonal banners line the main street of town, the colorful motifs changing with the celebrations of each season. It is a perfect town for long walks, movies, decent shopping, and most importantly, good restaurants. Pasadena is so civilized the trash men collect the garbage in tiny little trucks that come right up the driveway to pick up your trash. You never have to remember garbage day in Pasadena. If you are a local, you frequently don't need to show a driver's license to cash a check, and Baskin Robbins will run a tab for you.

I had spent one year of my life in Pasadena before nursing school. That was enough to permanently endear the town to me. Sam was a young attractive man, straddling the threshold of the closet. He hadn't decided how far out he wanted to come as a gay man. The West Side was perfect for Sam. West Hollywood, Santa Monica, Beverly Hills, Westwood, Venice Beach, and Malibu are whatever is cool, hot, or bad, at the moment. That means at this very moment, because Bad is an extremely transient, elusive thing. When it's on the West Side at Spagos it's hot, by the time it makes it over to the Valley its boring. To live as God intended a West Sider to live, you have to make the effort to be in the know. Slow in the know does not count, life is too fast here for that. I'm slow. By the time I'd heard of Wolfgang Puck, he was getting ready to open a chain of Puck Burgers in the Valley.

Someone who is really cool makes it look effortless. How do they get their information? Are there hotlines, magazines, secret code words? As close as Sam and I became, I never understood how he knew just what he knew. I realized back in junior high that God had given some people the gift of being cool. Some girls appear to have been born knowing where to buy Erase, and Maybelline's Midnight Blue mascara. The cool belong on the West Side. They gravitate there and revel in the trendy moment. That's one of the reasons I like the East Side. Its quiet, understated, elegant. Trends shift slowly there; I can keep up with them.

Sam and I introduced one another to our turfs. I took him to movies, dinners, and gracious luncheons in Pasadena. None of this blew his socks off. He was polite, but not enchanted. I was more successful with Evelyn. I even converted her to the Pasadena life for a few years. But Sam wanted more motion, more life, more intensity. He told me he would take us dancing at his favorite club, Circus Circus. I was excited, this was great. I was going clubbing with a cool West Sider.

Clubbing is not easy. You don't go near a club until eleven at the earliest and I usually go to bed at ten. One. So I took a nap, but it was hard to sleep because I was too excited. I called Sam to see what he was wearing. The Uniform- tight jeans, perfect white shirt, sleeves rolled up, narrow black leather tie. I didn't have a cool uniform, so I fussed and worried about my clothes, hair and make-up for a couple of hours. At ten thirty I went down to his room in my tightest jeans, a pretty blouse and dancing shoes. It was hard to confuse me with Cinderella as I climbed into Sam's green V.W. bug. But I was hopeful, excited, and up way past my bedtime.

I don't know what I was really thinking this evening would be like. I had pictures of Sam and I dancing all night while viewing exotic looking people. We might even talk to cool people, make new friends. A whole new social world might be opening up for me. I hadn't really taken into consideration that I was going to a trendy gay club, with a gay man. Somehow I held a fantasy of myself in an intense conversation with Cher and Barbra Streisand; I would probably become deeply involved with William Hurt.

Not looking at things very clearly seems to have been a trait of mine. I find myself reluctant to ask basic questions. With whom am I dealing? What does their behavior tell me about them? What does my behavior tell me about me?

The last question I am particularly slow to explore. If I had asked myself any of these questions, I would have given up on the picture of William and I, intensely engaged in conversation and tea at two a.m. I am not a social butterfly, I am more like a quiet observer. The likelihood of Sam spending all evening dancing with me, when he was surrounded by the best looking males the West Side had to offer was slim. And, in reality, I knew Cher probably had other plans that evening.

Whatever glitz and glamour I had prepared myself to see, I was not prepared for Circus, Circus. We parked about a block away, where it was free, and said good-by to our valuables locked in Sam's glove compartment. We entered Circus, and I was instantly blind in the darkness until my eyes could adjust. The place was dark and glittery. Well-muscled, naked chests were shoving through the crowd. These were the waiters in tight black pants, one arm extended high in the air, balancing a tray rimmed with tiny neon flashing lights.

Sam had told me about these waiters, and how great they looked. The waiters paled in comparison to the spectacle of their clients. Glistening sweaty flesh was everywhere. The view was mesmerizing. Farmer John overalls worn over nothing was one predominant theme. The men showed a little more anatomical insight than women frequently do. They tended to select their costume style by body type. The big beefy types stuck to the overalls and naked look, frequently leaving one side undone to show as much pumped up skin as possible. Slender beauties took more to the elegant or G.Q. look; Sam was of this ilk.

As I studied the crowd, patterns began to emerge in the chaos. I could see the aggressive men on the prowl. I saw the tentatively hopefuls, wondering if anyone special would notice them tonight. There were the young beautiful blondes, with bodies that would drive even Adonis to envy. The young and gorgeous strutted in, owning the world tonight. Once I got past the outrageous, sheer ballsy spectacle, I realized I had seen the underlying patterns before. It was the same thing, gay or straight; people searching for someone all look the same. The attitude seems to vary with how the individual perceives their chance of success.

I felt as if I were a child traveling through Circus with Sam. I hung on tight and eyeballed everyone in sight. The crowd was thick; while traversing the room an unseen hand groped my crotch. "Strange," I thought, "not titillating, and too impersonal to be considered flattery or effrontery, more along the lines of a gynecological exam."

These are scenes that probably can't be found anymore. The days of serious repercussions for flamboyant behavior are upon us. Our national focus is no longer on poverty, hunger, war, and racism. We have been told drugs and sex will lead our nation into darkness, so people must toe the line, at least publicly. I believe bad judgment, greed, and fearful thinking leads our nation into darkness, but no one of any importance has asked my opinion. As a social voyeur who enjoys glimpsing the bold and the outrageous, I am sorry about the current trend. Repression is rarely interesting to watch. The pendulum always swings; I look forward to the return of an interesting view in my old age.

The women at Circus Circus were in the minority. Some of them were there because they like hanging out with gay men. Some enjoyed the social liberation of the place. There were women here wild beyond what I thought people could be, in public or private. The most riveting for me was a trio of two women and a man. My eye was drawn to the three of them because they were wearing the shortest shorts on the face of the planet. The man wore only tiny shorts; the women wore bikini tops with theirs. They danced as a trio. The women's movements were so sexual I was hypnotized, until I recognized the man. He was a resident at County, a radiologist. We had talked once by the pool. He told me he liked radiology because he didn't have to interact with his patients much. He struck me as not interesting or bright, and I hoped I never ended up under his x-ray beam.

Later that evening I was to see him and his friends leave in a corvette with a personalized plate, "HOT DOC." Hot Doc may have lacked luster professionally, but his personal life was real strange. These three performed everything short of intercourse right there on the dance floor. It was dark, so I can't swear they stopped at that. Many of the gay men were erotic, and intensely sexual, but they couldn't touch this trio for sheer exhibitionism.

An exhibitionist needs an audience, and I admit I was transfixed. Sam had abandoned me to dance with Ronnie, his close friend. This left me pressed against a wall in a room where no man had any intention of dancing with me. I don't mind asking men to dance. I find it highly preferable to waiting to be asked. I did not get the feeling that any of these men would be open to my approach. I will dance with a girl friend; when circumstances allow women are great dancing partners. I never ask strange women to dance, and in this bar, strange took on a whole new meaning. So I watched Doc and his friends do unbelievable things to each other in a room crammed with people, where nobody paid any attention. This trio was a lot more inventive than anything I saw at the Kit Kat Club, and they were doing it for free.

I stood through an interminably long slow song while Sam held Ronnie gently, and Doc undulated and palpated his friends. Finally the tune changed, the beat picked up, and Sam graced me with a dance, while Ronnie pouted. I hadn't known Ronnie was going to be there that night. I also hadn't known he would be so unwilling to share Sam. Apparently Sam didn't know this either. Ronnie was five foot two, one hundred pounds, South American, and perfectly adorable, all the way down to his accent. He wore a pout like it had been tailored for him. I knew Sam was doomed. The pursed lips and sad eyes charmed him completely.

Sam and I began to dance. The floor was crowded, people were jammed together. I yelled in Sam's ear about Doc, I wanted to know if he recognized him. We maneuvered our way around the dance floor and ended up next to the trio. I angled my body to give Sam a good look and ended up side by side with Hot Doc. I looked over into bleary eyes that held no glimmer of recognition. I watched the trio and noticed that each dancer took turns doubling over and tucking their head into their chest for a moment. The head was then thrown back, eyes glazed, lips smiling. I couldn't figure it out. I asked Sam, "what are they doing?" "Poppers", he said.

Poppers; amyl nitrate, I remember. I asked Sam, "have you done poppers?" "No!" he shook his head. I should have figured this, Sam is like me, fascinated by the unusual, but not willing to take any real risks. Apparently, Hot Doc had never been lectured as a youth on "high risk, low gain behavior". He turned to me, foggy faced, and graciously offered me a hit on his popper bottle. The Miss Manners in me politely thanked him and declined.

This shit is bad, you inhale it, it rushes to your brain, fries all the circuitry, and dissipates in a matter of seconds. Before crack, it was the "wham, bam, thank-you Ma'am" of drugs. Poppers would run your entire body through the alarm state in a matter of seconds. They became popular to use right at the moment of orgasm, as if your body is not already in enough alarm during orgasm. I looked around the room and noted that Doc and his friends weren't the only ones boosting their sympathetic nervous systems a little.

Sam and I finally got sweaty enough to need a break. We looked for Ronnie, but his pout had exhausted him, and he had gone home. The hour was nearing two A.M., and I was lapsing into coma from lack of sleep, so we left. Our exit was timed perfectly with The Doc's. I squealed and woke up completely when I saw his license plate. I couldn't let it go, it was so perfect. I drove Sam nuts with variations on Hot Doc jokes until we were in his car and ready to go.

We decided to end our evening on a full stomach. We went to the New Orleans all night coffee shop for breakfast. Over french toast and eggs, Sam told me about his last visit here. He and Ronnie had breakfast, and then went upstairs to see a psychic. She read their palms, and basically told Sam to dump the little guy. Ronnie was not pleased, Sam was intrigued, and my faith in psychics was growing. As we talked, the lights in my head started slowly going out, one by one. Its an interesting feeling. I can feel my IQ. drop in increments as each word leaves my mouth. I was moving towards a walking coma. I am not a person who can push past fatigue and go on I come to a dead stop. Sam was not impressed with my lack of enduranc. We left before he had to carry me.

I am an excellent play pal until ten p.m., in a pinch I can push it to eleven or twelve. Friends that I have seduced out to play, have complained about this. Most learn to live with my limitations. Sam and I spent the majority of our time playing in the afternoons and evenings. He talked me into buying the highest heeled cowboy boots I have ever seen. I have nearly killed myself wearing them. I finally gave them to a friend who is into higher risk behaviors than I am.

Luckily, Sam and I were placed together in all our rotations for the rest of nursing school. Administration at County apparently noticed who was friends with whom, and kept them together. We had met in obstetrics, we went on to become confidants and true buds in pediatrics. I was the only person with whom Sam would attend a nursing school party, a major coup for me, and he got me back to Circus Circus one more time.

Chapter Nineteen

Lessons in Living

I wasn't sure how I would feel about my rotation on the pediatric unit. Sick children and babies effect people in different ways. Some of the student nurses walked around in their Mickey Mouse aprons glowing like Mother Theresa. There is that Madonna look (the original one) that some females have when caring for puppies and sick children. I have noticed this phenomenon is the strongest in unmarried females.

I don't think I display this nurturing glow when holding a child. I generally like children or not, depending upon their personalities and attitudes. This sometimes concerns me. What if I have no maternal instincts? Preparing to work on the pediatric ward was anxiety-provoking for those of us who weren't sure if we had the nurturing instinct. I never baby-sat as a teenager. I had my own baby sitter until I was eighteen.

When you worked pediatrics you were allowed to wear "colorful aprons" to put the children at ease. The girls either made or bought, who knows where, pinafore-type aprons. The patterns on these varied among cartoon characters, bright sunny flowers, and of course, happy faces. The aprons had big ruffles around the neck, over the shoulders and down the back. The waistband tied in the back in a huge bow. It was a baby's pinafore. I guess the thinking was, if you looked like a baby, you wouldn't frighten a baby.

Grown women always look ridiculous when they dress like children. Even as a child I knew this. Some females occasionally get an apparently overwhelming desire to dress in an infantile manner. They'll find an excuse to put on a costume that should have been retired a millennium ago. This may be related to the mating ritual, wanting the male species to see how cute they were as a child. If you missed it then, you can see it now. Or possibly, if they were pretty as a child, they will produce pretty children. I haven't figured it out. Maybe if I had perceived myself as an adorable child, or a darling teen, I too would experience these regressive desires. Fortunately, I feel I look better now than then. Otherwise, I too might have been prancing around in a pinafore. God knows, I am not above a little regressive behavior.

Our first day on Peds our instructor, Betty Thomas, walked us around, and showed us the ropes. Betty intimidated me a bit because she had a no-nonsense look about her. She was smart, serious and well-educated. Unlike our other instructors, Betty would have lunch with us. Frequently she, Sam, and I would eat together. This is when I got to know Betty a bit and grew to like her. She was a strong technical nurse and she wasn't ooie-gooie over babies. This was because she was normally an advanced medical/surgical nurse for the senior rotation. This was also why she intimidated me. Those instructors were known to be difficult.

My first patient on Peds was a three-month old baby, a little girl whose mother had decided to quiet her crying one night with cough syrup. The bottle was marked for adults and children over six years, but people seldom take warning labels on over the counter medications seriously. The assumption is, if it's sold in the supermarket, it can't really hurt you. It's a dangerous assumption. Several tablespoons throughout the evening had put this baby into a coma. She was semi-conscious now, and severely brain damaged. It was a sad situation. Sad for the baby, and worse for the mother.

All the information was on the baby's chart. Parental induced drug overdose incenses the staff, even if it is accidental. Everyone is sure they would never be so stupid as to do something like this to their baby. The causes for disasters like this are lack of education, poor judgment, immature parents, and possibly illiteracy, but it is still a tragic accident. The staffs' hearts were with the baby, not the mother. By the time I was assigned to little Ann, she had been in the hospital for a month and her mother had stopped coming to see her altogether. I was told by one nurse that she thought the mother felt too guilty and couldn't deal with facing the staff. I don't know, because I never saw Ann's mother or father during the week I took care of her.

Baby Ann was sweet and easy to care for Betty showed me how to hold her safely like a football in one arm while I changed her bed. Once I got the football carry down, taking care of Ann was a breeze. Unlike full grown patients, babies are tiny, clean, and easy to take care of. When the work of changing linens, cleaning, and feeding them is done, you get to hold and cuddle them all you want. Everyone on the unit walked around with a baby in their arms or a child on their hip. There were children to be played with and teased everywhere.

Peds is not a sad unit; its a noisy lively fun place. Most of the children will get well and go home. In the meantime they are still children, like puppies; you can't stop them from playing, so you might as well join in. Five year olds will play jokes and tricks on you that you have to search back to your five year old mind to understand. This doesn't mean that pediatrics is not a heartrending place. There are some very sick little kids here. Betty walked us through the intensive care unit filled with babies that would never be well.

We walked around frequently on Peds visiting the different rooms where students were assigned. There was an unhappy, plump, fussy little three-year-old girl who was as yellow as a daffodil. Her small face was so puffed up with edema, she could hardly open her eyes. She was all tears and unhappiness on Monday. She looked like a miniature fat old lady, dipped in yellow paint. I didn't like this child. I thought "Ugh, what a fussy, difficult kid to love." I was glad to have sweet little Ann as my charge. People were all over the little girl trying to console her, distract her and coddle her. I viewed these women as the all nurturing females who could cuddle anybody, no matter how unpleasant. To me, she looked like a spoiled fussy baby and I wanted nothing to do with her.

Two days latter, when we returned, the little yellow fussball had metamorphosed into a gregarious, squirming, laughing, uncontainable doll. Without the edema and yellow color, her expressions and smiles charmed us. Her nature was one of unbounding love for everyone. This was one of those nagging lessons in life that remind me I am not the person I would like to be. I am definitely not an all-loving saint. My first reaction to her change was to be grateful I hadn't fired off my mouth about how obnoxious a child she was.

Peds was full of emotional lessons on a daily basis. I would watch a friend care for a baby so sick, undersized and full of tubes that the baby had no possibility of ever achieving a healthy life, and I would return with relief to a seven year old girl with the measles. I would wonder how my friend could overcome revulsion and care for such a distorted child. Sure as anything, the next week that baby was assigned to me, and it was my turn to learn more about love.

My teacher was the mother, Laura, who walked into the room and lit up with smiles of delight each morning when she saw her daughter. She explained to me how Michelle had been born with water on the brain and required an operation immediately after her birth. The fluid still continued to build up, requiring frequent operations. Michelle was nearly eighteen months old and she was the size of a six month old infant. Laura told me of Michelle's bravery and courage. How excited she had been when a few weeks ago Michelle sat up for the first time by herself.

This mother's pride was as pronounced as if her daughter had just graduated college. Laura may have been even prouder than the mother of the normal child who accomplishes a normal feat like graduating, Michelle had done the extraordinary, she sat up. Laura taught me the in's and out's of Michelle. She explained which of Michelle's behaviors were brand new and which ones were landmarks of progress along the way. Laura didn't talk about what her daughter would some day be, or some day do. She celebrated in the moment the fact that Michelle could curl her fingers around her hand, a skill recently acquired.

The excitement and love were infectious. By the second day I had learned to be more observant to the little signs of Michelle's delight or frustration. The feelings and moods were all present in this little one. You just had to get quiet and pay attention or you would miss the subtle details of Michelle and that would be a shame, because by then she had me. I had finally seen her through the mess of tubes, and loved her. I have always recognized and honored the infinite possibilities in life. Michelle and her mother helped me touch and appreciate the finite.

My last set of lessons on pediatrics took place with Tommy as my teacher. I walked in on Friday to check next week's assignment so I could work up a major care plan over the weekend. I was too busy playing with Sam earlier in the rotation, so I had to do my big care plan on my last patient. I saw Tommy and thought great, this kid looks good. He was five years old and bouncing around in bed with a huge smile. This is gonna be a breeze. I read his chart and wrote down all the important information I would need to research his case for my care plan.

I went to my medical text book and looked up Tommy's diagnosis, astrocytoma. He had a fast growing, malignant brain tumor. I felt like a box came crashing down over my head, closing me in. I had seen what I had wanted to see, a happy kid; what I had was a dying child.

I timidly entered Tommy's room on Monday. I need not have been timid. The room was so full of people and noise that no one noticed me for a few moments. Tommy was the center of attention, sitting up and taking turns banging everybody on the head with his new doll, Chewbacca. Those receiving the blows were his mother, stepfather, the head nurse on the unit, and his intern. I was recognized as a new head to be banged. His mother quickly noticed that I was wearing a nursing cap, and a bang would do it no good. I told Tommy I was his nurse this week and he could thwap me on the arm instead. I then held my arm out to make it convenient for him. Pow, Chewbacca had now conquered me too. Tommy was triumphant.

His tired mother smiled at me apologetically. "I know we spoil him, and that's not good for him, but it's so hard to say no when he wants something." I had no reply. I smiled and told her it was OK, Chewie was my favorite character in Star Wars. I was accepted as part of the team; we were all here to take care of Tommy. His stepfather told me that when Tommy was diagnosed they took him to Toys-R-Us, and told him to take his pick. He could have any toy he wanted. They were prepared to do it right, even a bike if he wanted. But Tommy had just seen the movie, and he wanted Chewie. I got the sense it had been a little frustrating for the stepfather. There is very little guilt release in buying a ten dollar doll. Adults tend to feel guilty around dying children; it all seems so unfair.

This was a room full of guilty adults, all trying to make little Tommy happy even though he's dying. At the center of them all Tommy sat manipulating the crowd with five year old nonsense. People were so busy trying to deal with his antics that the real life struggle for his life became eclipsed, until necessity thrust it forward. It was time for his medication. Tommy's tumor caused swelling in his brain, giving him an unbearable headache. The medications were to decrease the swelling. Unfortunately, most meds have side effects, and this one made him nauseous. Sometimes the nausea was severe enough to cause vomiting, which increased the pain in his head terribly.

Though only five, Tommy had put everything together, pill, barf, blinding headache, and was refusing to take his meds. His mother coaxed him to the point of tears, hers. His stepfather, angry frustrated, and in his own pain, threatened and tried to force him to take the pill, to the point of tears, Tommy's. I watched, trying not to fall into the vortex of pain with the rest of them. We knew if Tommy kept crying his headache would increase to the point where we wouldn't have medication to contain it without knocking him out. You don't want to snow a five year old with terminal cancer.

I couldn't stand it any longer. I asked them all to stop and to let me try. I took Tommy's medication, and told him to be quiet and relax. I would try to fix the pill and make it better. It had occurred to me that a capsule opening past the stomach in the small intestine should not make him nauseous. I ground the pill into a fine powder. I then carefully scooped it up with a little knife into an empty gelatin capsule, and closed it up. I returned to Tommy's room and sat on the bed. I asked if the two of us could be alone so we could talk.

Once we were alone the room became quiet, and Tommy looked at me with tears still running down his eyes. He was no longer a spoiled boy pushing everyone around, he was in pain and frightened about even worse pain. I told him I understood about the pills, and didn't want his stomach to be sick. I knew how much that hurt him. This was a better pill to help the pain. Tommy continued to cry, tearing at my heart, but I stayed together. I said "Tommy, I wouldn't give you this if I thought it would make you sick. I believe this pill will be better, and will help you. Trust me, take the pill."

I couldn't have sworn that the pill would be better. I was only a student nurse, not a pharmacist. It made sense, but it was an easy solution, if it was good, why hadn't somebody thought about it before? I was only doing my best, but I couldn't promise him anything. I was asking a dying child in pain to trust me, when my faith in myself was delicate and tentative.

I had looked into his eyes. I had said it with my heart. Tommy took the pill. I thanked him, kissed him, and laid him down to rest. Outside the door his mother and stepfather were waiting, they had been listening. His mother told me I was going to make a wonderful nurse, I thanked her. I made it back to the medication room and closed the door, before I was overcome with sobs. The pain vortex had gotten me, and swallowed me completely.

Tommy was my patient for the rest of the week. The capsules were effective, the medication no longer made him nauseous. I spent all my time with Tommy and his mother. We went everywhere together. He especially liked the ride to his radiation treatment. He would put on his P.J.'s and a robe, and then we would wrap him in a hospital blanket, like an Indian. We carried him down to the basement where we would wait for the electric cart to come for us. We would climb onto the cart, give the driver our destination, and Tommy would tell him to "go real fast". We then became hell on wheels. Unlike the normal mother who becomes anxious when her child is driven in a reckless manner, this woman was just glad to see her's happy and alive.

We would careen along on a wild ride through the tunnels underlying County. I had never been down there before, and the ride was exciting. The tunnels were just wide enough for two vehicles to pass each other, if nobody stuck out a finger. Big, electric hospital beds were left abandoned here and there, along with all kinds of unidentifiable stuff. You never knew what you would come upon around the next corner. Our driver would honk his horn and whirl around a corner like an Indy driver. Tommy would laugh and egg him on.

We would finally arrive at the location for radiation patients. Here Tommy would get quiet. He hated being put in the huge, tube-like structure. Tommy's head was slid into what looked like a large front loading washing machine. He was told to hold absolutely still on a cold hard table, while everyone left the room. We watched from behind a thick lead window while Tommy's head was irradiated. So far this form of treatment had shown no statistical improvement on cancers like his. But in the face of such impotence, doctors and parents have to do something. If there was a minute possibility it might help, it had to be tried.

The boy we retrieved from the big scary machine was not the one we had placed in it. This Tommy was exhausted, feeling ill, and frightened. This was a baby needing his mother. She held him wrapped in the blanket while we waited for our ride back. The same driver would pick us up. The ride back was slow and careful and quiet.

When we weren't in the throws of emotional trauma, it was easy to forget he was a very sick boy. Tommy looked like any devilish, somewhat spoiled, five year old. He hadn't lost his hair, like many do with chemotherapy. His type of cancer was not responsive to this treatment; it was also inoperable because of the location. The books say two to three years is the lifespan expected of patients with Tommy's type of malignant tumor. The average is fifty-two weeks after diagnosis. Fifty-two weeks didn't seem like much time.

I don't know how long Tommy lived. The rest of his life was going to be spent in and out of County. He was becoming a regular, and a staff pet. His death would leave a void at County, in the hearts of the nurses and the staff that had worked with him. The void would be partially, and sadly, filled by the next terminally ill child, who would live out their short, painful life in and out of the halls at County. You also miss the families, mothers and fathers that no longer have a reason to come in and chat with you, people with whom you share an intense emotional time, lives overlapping. Then, they are gone. This isn't unique to pediatrics; it is intrinsic to nursing. Lives are brought together when everything is up in the air, and the balance in the scales is changing. No wonder I would sometimes feel more intimacy in my work life than off duty. When emotions are raw, people are more open with one another.

Nursing school was a sequence of lessons I needed to learn, I just hadn't known what the curriculum would be. I had lost my fear of pediatrics. I had gained a new respect for the staff there and for myself. This wasn't an overwhelming, life changing, new sense of self. It was a subtle knowledge that I could do more than I had thought, handle things that I had assumed would undo me. I realized that this was true for most people. Nurses in pediatrics may be special people. But it is a matter of choice, not a gift from the Gods. It is important for me to know my decisions are a matter of choice, and not a series of personal limitations.

Pediatrics gave me a sense of how much I enjoyed working with children. It also taught me that no matter how delightful my patients were I still did not care for the physical aspects of nursing. My list of possible options for a career in nursing was getting shorter with each rotation. My final rotation in 201 was Psychiatry. I looked forward to Psych as my last hope for a clean form of nursing where creative thinking was more important than sterile technique.

Chapter Twenty

Romance Redeux

I was beginning to feel restless. I had recovered from the trauma of disengaging from Michael and was entering an area of nursing I was excited about, Psychiatry. I had also passed a plateau in school. With only six months of school left I was over the hump of the halfway point. Real life was out there waiting for me. Though I knew my hardest clinical courses lay ahead of me at this point, I figured I was going to graduate, life would go on, and I would be expected to nurse.

It became very clear to me what I was in the mood for: romance. I wasn't looking for an intense, wild fling. I was ready to fall in love. Just like that. It seemed the timing was perfect. I was available. I wanted to be deeply involved, with someone to take seriously as a life partner. I wanted that fresh injection of energy into my life that comes with a new love. But I didn't want something temporary. I wasn't looking for much, just a life-long partner who could match me stride for stride. As contemporary as I wanted to be, in my heart I wanted what my mother and father have, life long love, still holding hands and kissing at seventy.

I was amazed at Evelyn's honesty in announcing her ideal timeline. She wanted to fall in love first semester with the perfect man. They would be engaged by the end of our first year, and get married after graduation. They would have their first baby within the next year. Her description was so blunt and contrived, I couldn't believe she would give it voice, even to me.

I knew that is not how it goes. Love can't be planned, it must be magic. If you announce your desires, you are sure to drive them away. Besides, what man wants to get involved with a woman who is scheming for marriage? I spouted off to Evelyn some pack of lies about career, focusing on myself rather than on a man, all intelligent stuff; in my heart, I thought her timeline sounded perfect. Evelyn's statement was too on the mark, too painfully accurate. I lied to her; more confounding, I lied to me.

So here I was within six months of graduation, and finally ready to admit, at least to myself, that I wanted a mate. I decided I was ready to try dating, an area where I had little experience. I was ready to meet new people (marriageable men), and this seemed the traditional way to do it.

There is no reason I shouldn't date. I don't have a third leg or drool much. However, I never really got the hang of acquiring a date. My flirting skills are weak. I could never find the right dial to control my flirting output. Too much flirt, and every hound dog in the vicinity is howling. Too little flirt, and you have what I have, no dates. My mother told me when I was fourteen that I needed to be nicer to boys, that I wasn't doing it right. She told me flirting was an art and any girl could do it. For some reason I was resistant. I thought my behavior was admirable. I don't connive and flirt. I am outspoken and honest. I think the real reason had to do with fear of rejection. What a bummer to put all that energy into being coy and seductive, while seeing his eyes follow a petite brunette as she crosses the room.

I was ready, though I wasn't sure how to begin. I could pin a note to my chest saying, "I know I have been aloof and unreceptive to any advances in the past. But, I am now ready to begin social dating for the purpose of finding my perfect mate." I hadn't told any one yet that I wanted to date, but I was definitely thinking about possible ways to approach the situation. This is when Jeff intervened.

Jeff and I had stayed consistently good friends and lovers through out nursing school. We had been seeing each other almost weekly for over a year. We mostly talked about who we were seeing and how we felt about them. We also talked frequently about Jeff's work. He was a graphic artist, just branching out, and starting his own company. We talked about his approach to work, what type of company he wanted to create for himself. We combed through the in's and out's of his daily experiences at the office.

I don't remember us talking about nursing much. Nursing is something like being a cop, or in the military. Its sort of an in-group, out-group kind of thing. If you do it, you talk about it, sometimes constantly. If you don't do it, you probably don't want to hear about it. I could tell this because as I would talk about a difficult day on the wards Jeff's eyes would glaze over and fade away. He would also absent-mindedly change the topic back to his work if I paused too long taking a breath.

This lack of reciprocity concerning interest in each other's careers bothered me. I felt boring and unheard. I didn't get too carried away about it though. Unless someone is a doctor or a nurse, they usually have a low tolerance for hospital talk. I have also noted, it is the rare man who can produce as much interest in my career as I can whip up over his. I like business. I grew up in a home where dinnertime conversation was frequently focused on business. I was excited about Jeff's tiny new company. I would listen to him tirelessly, give him my best advice, make suggestions. I didn't do this out of sweetness or love. I did it out of sheer enjoyment of the process. I wasn't the only one interested in Jeff's career. He told me over Mexican food that an old girlfriend had just returned from Australia. She had recently surprised him at his office.

His eyes sparkled and his face became animated as he described his past relationship to Peggy. Of course she was absolutely beautiful. Has there ever been a past girlfriend who wasn't? They had enjoyed an intense affair. They had been two highly driven career types, managing to make time for some steamy sex. This is probably not a fair description, but I had to glean what I could from Jeff's rose-colored memories. One thing was clear, the heat had not cooled down. Jeff and Peggy were in that tantalizing place of "would they or wouldn't they."

A beautiful, high-intensity, driven woman in Jeff's life didn't thrill me. I would pale by comparison, and probably get much less of his attention. Peggy wanted them to "work" together. She was into public relations, he was a commercial artist. She had the drive and ability to move his career forward. My irritation at all this was mild, but grating. I felt like a lioness who's territory was being invaded. What probably bothered me the most was that my dear friend had gone and found true love when he wasn't looking for it, while I floundered in how to search for a mate.

I spent the next month or so hearing how Jeff and Peggy were going to work together without getting involved. Both wanted only a professional connection. Right. I gave them one or two more weeks of that nonsense at the most. I didn't buy this platonic act and I told Jeff, "It is just a matter of time". He told me I was wrong, and I heard echoes of myself, saying the same thing about Michael. I think this is based on the principal of the human eyeball - it is built to look outward, not inward. For me, looking inward takes an act of courage, and force.

I was busy myself during these weeks attempting to be outgoing. I must not have looked very natural in the process. People didn't seem to quite trust me as an outgoing person. Something was off. I felt awkward and uneasy., but couldn't figure out what the problem was. I still don't know what I was emanating on encountering men. Fear, desperation, or maybe my underlying boredom was seeping through to the surface; and they could smell it.

Before I ever really swung into action on my search for the perfect mate, Jeff surprised me again. He told me his friendship with me was interfering with his progressing in a relationship with Peggy. He and Peggy had made it past the "we just want to work together" stage. They had moved into "we think it may be love." Peggy was now looking for more of a commitment from Jeff. She was perfect for him, beautiful, work-oriented, great in bed, but he kept thinking about me.

We had never tried to move our connection to a primary relationship. One or the other of us was usually romantically involved with some other person. We had now been close friends for about three years. Jeff said he couldn't move forward with someone else while he still wondered about he and I. Would we be the perfect couple? I had my doubts. I had been wanting to fall in love with someone brand new, someone who's weakness and strengths lay out there yet to be discovered.

Jeff was like my favorite pair of jeans. Relationships and clothes have many things in common. There are your wonderful old outfits that feel great and look good every time you put them on. There are exciting new combinations, a little risqué and of questionable fit, but the feeling is exhilarating. If I am in the mood for a brand new outfit, a totally different look, it is hard to get worked up over an old favorite. Thus the syndrome "I have nothing in my closet to wear."

Nothing I own will make me feel the way I want to feel tonight. I need something new.

Needing a whole new look is similar to a hair attack. It is usually brought on by a sense of dissatisfaction with myself or my life. I was frightened by the realization that nursing school was coming to an end. On what would I focus? Around what force would my life revolve? A career in nursing would bring in money and keep me busy for eight hours a day, but that was not going to be enough. County and school were a way of life. Many County nurses never leave. They graduate from the School of Nursing, and go on to work at the hospital for the rest of their careers.

I didn't see myself following in this pattern. The only force I could picture strong enough to keep my life revolving in a cohesive manner was a man. I wanted a pivotal point like my mother had, something to form my life around. I looked for a man to come in and fill the vacuum in my life. Somehow in twenty-five years I had not collected enough of myself to trust that what I needed in the center of me, was me. Without knowing it, Jeff was asking for trouble. He was asking for the chance to fill my void, a gap badly needing filling by myself.

Jeff was clear in the direction he thought we should move. We should begin serious dating, for the purpose of deciding if we wanted to be together as mates. This way we would know once and for all if we were meant to be together. I had conflicting feelings to this piece of information, neither of which was very noble or romantic. I felt flattered and smug that the perfect Peggy was being put on hold for me. My intelligence and humor had won out over her perfection, making it all the more magical that he would want me. My other feeling was one of frustration. I didn't want to "fall in love" with Jeff. That did not sound exciting. I had found our conversations rather dull lately. I had been ready to strike out and explore new territory, not re-examine familiar terrain. So my response was, "fine". This way we can decide once and for all if we are romantically inclined to one another, and get on with our lives. I was pretty sure that we would discover that we were best as friends and romance for each of us should take place elsewhere.

One of our first dates under this new format was to the Ice House, a comedy club in Pasadena. Things got slow and the comic resorted to one of my most dreaded, bad comic tools, asking the audience dumb questions. "Any body out there from Wichita, what about that flat state of Kansas, huh?" Our comic moved on to focus on love. "Who out there is in love?" "Who's here with their best girl?" Jeff raised his hand and waved it in the air, smiling broadly. He's in love, he's here with his best girl. He gave me a squeeze to include me in his participatory excitement. I smiled, but it was tentative and cautious. I couldn't make the shift that fast. I wasn't sure at all about being in love. Loving someone and being in love are different.

Jeff and I had been very careful in the past not to cloud our friendship with the trappings of romance. We never made future plans together. We were careful not to lead each other into false impressions. We avoided romantic endearments. Not more than two weeks ago, Peggy had been the most incredible woman Jeff knew. Now, here I was, his best girl. I felt rushed. I wondered about the sincerity and depth of his feelings. However, I never said a word to him about any of it. I just let the uncomfortable moment pass.

I didn't want to confront the issue of my desire to fall in love with someone new. I didn't want to have to explore my feelings with Jeff. I didn't know what I would find. So I couldn't exactly push him to explore his. I was more comfortable with silent muddle than open confusion. In retrospect, I am sure open confusion would have been best. Chances are Jeff had some confusion of his own. We might have felt much more like friends exploring what was frightening to us, than the reticent romancers we were.

Jeff talked about marriage, and what was important to him. His wife must be a career woman. I must focus on my career and he would focus on his. We would be the perfect self-actualized team, knowing what we wanted and going for it. Certainly children were on the agenda two to three years down the road. For the moment though, we were to focus on our careers and build our lives. This would be music to many a woman's ears - a man who recognized and supported her need to achieve. I think I was over eating a hot fudge banana split when the need to achieve was being handed out to babies, and so I missed it.

I tried to explain this to Jeff. I had a small income. I wasn't looking to make a great deal of money, and I didn't want to work that hard. I didn't want to drive and push, achieve and succeed. I would rather spend my time with family and friends than out getting ahead in the world. It wasn't an issue of capability, it was a matter of drive and desire. This conflicted with Jeff's picture of his future mate. He had pictures of going to business dinners with a high powered woman by his side.

I decided the whole conversation was moot, who knew where this relationship was going. Jeff was a workaholic, his time with me was very limited. I told him I refused to discuss marriage with him until we had spent seventy-two consecutive hours together. He agreed this was reasonable. I figured I had increased our chances of taking a vacation together considerably. Besides, I couldn't seriously consider marrying anyone who won't chill out and take a decent vacation.

Jeff and I continued seeing each other on a regular basis. We would usually get together on Friday and Saturday evenings and frequently on Sunday. We went out to movies, inexpensive restaurants, or cooked at his place. We spent the weekend nights at his apartment. Weeks, and then months went by with my enjoying our time together, taking for granted that I would be with Jeff.

My father was turning sixty-five, and Mother was throwing him a surprise party at their country club. This was wonderful because I finally had a date normal enough to take to a serious party. After my eclectic collection of "interesting" looking men, Jeff was perfect. He was a six foot one, one hundred and ninety pound weightlifter. I could actually wear high heels. This was only partially wonderful because I can't walk one city block in heels; but standing totally still, with my hand gently holding on to an arm for balance, the effect is great. Jeff was also an artist with conservative, impeccable taste in clothes. He was a primper to the max, every hair in place, shoes freshly shined, nails buffed. This was a big change from a floor length wool cape and a felt fedora hat on a five foot four Michael.

Jeff always dressed in a more socially appropriate manner than I did. The man had his jeans laundered with heavy starch so the creases were perfect. It took the strength of a body builder just to pry them apart so he could insert his legs. I launder my jeans with two extra softener sheets in the dryer, so they are comfy to the point of limp. Attempting to look half as good as Jeff was a challenge.

I was very excited about dressing for this party. I had just had my twenty-seventh birthday. I felt mature enough, and my date looked sophisticated enough for me to finally own, and wear, a sexy dress. Having the nerve to own a sexy outfit and to wear one are two different things. I was ready to go to this party looking like a full grown, attractive, woman. Many females have this look at eighteen. I feel I finally crossed over into looking full grown at thirty-six. Its a good thing because soon I will be a "mature" woman and its nice to have made it to full grown first.

I went out shopping for a dress to die for. I was prepared to spend more money than usual. I was willing to spend up to seventy-five dollars. I was looking for sophisticated, classy, and sexy, which meant no red sequins, no fringe, no sparkles. I tramped around the mall for hours, feeling as though I were on maneuvers in the army. My mission had become an obsession. I searched until I found the perfect dress, a dream come true. It was silk, in that beautiful shade of blue that moves almost to lavender until you can't tell exactly what color it is. Sleeveless, it had a deep "V" neck with teal piping, and a reversible teal belt. The best thing about the dress was that it was slit up both sides, almost to the top of my thighs. I looked perfectly respectable, and felt totally sensual.

Whether or not you wear a bra makes a big difference in how clothes feel. Silk on bare breasts is one of the most sensual experiences one can have while fully dressed in public. This dress slipped over my body like a soft breath. When I moved, the slits flowed in the breeze of my stride, revealing my legs. Either the rest of the world was missing what I knew - that this was the perfect dress - or there had been a mistake. The price on the dress was half of what I was prepared to spend. I didn't think twice. I whipped out my check book and I owned it. I found some pale gray sandals with heels low enough that I could walk and dance in them. The party couldn't be soon enough.

I came home from the stores ready to unload my loot, and display it to Susan and Evelyn. My excitement was uncontainable. My enthusiasm far outweighed what was merited by even the most wonderful of dresses. Evelyn picked up on my overenthusiastic state of mind first, "You seem awfully excited about this date." Susan scrutinized my face, "It's true, you're glowing." Susan's look and tone made me feel like a Doris Day clone as she announced, "You're in love!" "That's it," Evelyn confirmed, "she's in love". Both of them stood there looking pleased and smug, as if they had just discovered a new disease of the week.

"No," I thought, "not with Jeff." Then, "Yes, why not? It's true." How does this happen? Do we really fall in love like this, one day noticing our feelings have changed? Or is the thought of being in love so spectacular we go with the suggestion? Did I re-arrange my feelings to embrace and maintain the moment? I could feel the blood rushing to my face a red hot flush of emotion. The reality was confirmed, "Look at her blush, she's in love."

Maybe it was true, I certainly wasn't sure yet. But it was exactly what I wanted. The timing was perfect. I smiled as I thought about it. There was nothing to be done, just wait and see. However, as I waited, I observed myself wearing an extra glow, an extra heavy dose of love songs running through my head.

The night finally arrived. I set aside two hours to get ready. Dressing can take me anywhere from five minutes to two and a half hours depending on time available, how foolish I'm feeling, and how hungry I am. Hunger speeds up the process immensely. I showered, then I curled my hair, then I wished I hadn't. This is a ritual with me. I decide I should curl my hair. This takes twenty to thirty minutes. My hair never curls in moderation. I look in the mirror to face a wild head of irregular, uncontrollable curls, and wonder why I did it. I think I do it to consume time when I am excited to go somewhere. It then takes another twenty minutes to contain the curls.

Curls minimally controlled, make-up on, sparkle shine panty hose (that run when you look at them, cost twelve dollars, and you have to carry two spare pairs) delicately pulled on, pits powdered and re-powdered at least seven times, I was so excited. I finally put on my beautiful silk dress. Now that I was dressed, I couldn't sweat one more drop for the rest of the evening. This is unrealistic, so for the short term I stuffed Kleenex under my arms while I waited for Jeff to call, announcing his arrival at my dorm.

Jeff had arrived. I walked down the hall to the elevator with my silk dress flipping open almost up to my panties. My dress exposed far too much leg to wear a slip without it showing. I was carefully brought up that a lady never allows her undergarments to show. Better a bit of skin, than a shot of a bra strap or a slip. Tonight I was displaying about eight feet of leg, but no lingerie.

The ballroom was already filling with people when Jeff and I entered. The guest of honor was due to arrive in twenty minutes. My eyes immediately searched for my sisters. In social settings we tend to flock together, enjoying each other's company the most. Because of this, Mother had been rigorous in separating the family for dinner, each daughter and her partner would be seated at a different table for dinner. This would ensure appropriate mingling.

I was delighted to be sitting between two great men, Jeff and an old family friend. Tonight felt magical, Jeff seemed to love everything about me. He spoke with pride regarding our relationship. "Yes", he agreed with my parents' friends, he was a very lucky man. In the glow of the evening's wine, and Jeff's admiration, I felt totally confident and at ease. The music began and it was time to dance. Jeff was a wonderful dancer. He had won prizes in competitions and took pride in his skill. Sometimes it tested his patience dancing with me. I am undisciplined, I move around from beat to counter-beat. Jeff had moves, great moves. I was all loose, with my hips sliding to the music. I think he felt I was not enhancing the look of his moves.

Jeff could get very testy with my dancing, but not tonight. Tonight I was perfect, and I loved it. My body snaked to the music, my dress slid up and open around my legs, and Jeff glowed. I was in heaven. Father came to take my hand for a fast dance. This is the man who taught me to dance. While Mother cooked, we would all take turns in our large kitchen, dancing with Daddy to the tune of Mack the Knife. Finally one of us would be assigned to watch the cheese bread for burning, while Mother took over the floor with Father. These two can dance; they own the floor and you can feel the energy crackle between them.

I am always a little nervous when Father asks me to dance. I don't want to disappoint him. I am also excited, he was the first man I danced with, and the thrill has never dimmed. I didn't want to goof up. The band was good, I was feeling full of myself, head back, fanny out, we danced away. As he led me back to my seat next to Jeff, Father said, "I didn't know you could dance." The comment struck me funny. I was delighted at his notice, but I wondered what ever made him think I couldn't?

Throughout the evening as I made trips to the ladies' room, I would be approached by my mother's friends. They told me what a great looking man Jeff was, he seemed like such a nice person. "You girls always find the handsome men." Jeff reported to me his experience in the men's room was similar. I was beautiful, he was truly lucky. I always wonder about comments like this. What if I were a beautiful bitch, would he still be lucky?

Tonight I was thankful that stress had not mangled my complexion, and my hair was not too wild or weird. My hair couldn't get too wild because Jeff had taken over cutting it. He had studied it for awhile, given it some thought and then taken his scissors to it. Punk was in. If I were going to be cool, which Jeff hoped I would be, my hair had to be somewhat punk. I wasn't up for a radical look. I wouldn't let him bleach it and dye it pink, but I let him get it pretty short. The front was supposed to stand straight up, which it would do only for him. So the curlers I had forced into my short hair could create only so much havoc. My hair was as short as a boy's in back, and tonight the top was curly.

Through out our years together, I gave my head over to Jeff. He became quite skilled at cutting, frosting, and perming. He usually kept me looking clean, sharp, and classic. My wardrobe took on preppie overtones, with a heavy dose of blazers and vests. I enjoyed his involvement in my appearance. I felt the love and caring in his attention. I also felt the critical eye he used to assess me, the need for padding around my chest, and weight lifting to build up my arms. His feelings about appearances made the comments of others at the party especially reassuring. I was given a stamp of approval. Of course, I can't imagine my parents' friends finding me anything but delightful; after all they are their friends. I was also reassured my choice of men was wonderful, that this man was a gem. Somehow the nod of approval from the general populace was very reassuring for both Jeff and me. If I was still feeling a little shaky in my own judgment of this relationship, it was comforting to know others thought my choice was a sound one.

It was a long evening, with another hour-long drive to Jeff's apartment. We were both numb with fatigue by the time we reached his front door. The warm feelings we shared at the party had lasted even through the exhaustion. We replayed all our favorite parts of the evening, and then went to sleep feeling loving and confident in the warm reception we had received as a couple.

The glow did not dim with the morning light. My mind and body decided they liked this new state just fine. I was looking for love and romance, and here it was. The timing was right, I was ready, what a delight. We would be a couple, we would make plans and move forward. This was love! The glow spread from my head, took root in my stomach, and began to fire my life with a new light. I was a woman in love, Jeff was my mate. Once again my life had focus and meaning. Graduation did not loom so large on the horizon to frighten me, because I had Jeff to stand beside me. When anxieties are high, and life seems scary and unpredictable, romance is the best salve I know. I welcomed Jeff and our love into my heart with open arms, and embraced them.

Chapter Twenty-One

"You Must Conceptualize"

I was nervous and excited as I took a seat in the classroom. I had been looking forward to Psychiatric Nursing for almost two years. It was my last hope for finding a form of nursing that didn't make me want to lose my breakfast. Psych was perfect; clean, nothing oozes or drips and people's entrails stayed where they belonged, on the inside, where I wouldn't have to deal with them. It sounded great, no bed pans, no I.V.'s, and best of all, no uniforms. For three brief months I would be released from the confines of that God-awful dress County made us wear.

I should be good at psych. I was the psychosocial nurse. I loved helping people sort out their problems. I was not afraid to give advice. I could recommend a sane course of action. And, I was, of course, incredibly mentally healthy. I had no fears of undiscovered mental illness, phobias, or neurosis lurking inside me. There is something scary about working with psychiatric patients. The inner workings of the mind gone awry are unnerving. For some it is just a little unnerving, for others it is totally unacceptable. It is almost impossible not to question one's own grip on reality and inner lines of communication, when dealing with people who have chosen such alternative ways of living inside their head.

I should be good at this. That's why I was so nervous. After a year and a half in nursing school, telling everyone and myself, that I was going to major in psych the pressure was on. I was worried because I didn't have another ace in the hole. Psych was it, it was the only nursing slot I could see myself fitting into. My bachelor's degree is in psych, and I am the most verbal person God ever put on the planet. I should be able to do this.

Flo Davidson was the instructor who would evaluate our competence in psychiatric nursing. This did not soothe my fears. Flo is wild, boisterous, flamboyant, assertive, confrontational and extremely blunt. She is smart and knowing in that shrewd way nature gave us at birth. She has the kind of truth sensors that the school systems spend years trying to eradicate. To sweet, nice, normal people, Flo is clearly crazy. When I saw Flo, I thought of Tom Wolfe's reflections on Marshal McCluen and wondered, "What if she is right?"

Any student at County knew of Flo long before he or she took her class. Flo Davidson, RN. is a visual phenomenon. She is a large black woman somewhere in the middle of her life, with a buxom, well-proportioned figure. Her shoulder length hair was perfectly jerri-curled. Flo had style. She walked into a room with an explosion of color: a scarf at her neck, bright red come-fuck-me pumps on her feet. She was not very stable on her high heels because her vision was rapidly failing from years of fighting diabetes. The onset of blindness frustrated the hell out of her, but she charged ahead, dominating all the space surrounding her.

Flo was a grabber. If she wanted to talk to you, she would grab your arm in a firm grip so she knew she had your attention. The Davidson Clinch may have been a more recently acquired trait, a compensation for a diminishing ability to maintain strong eye contact. If she could no longer penetrate you with her eyes, she could hold you in her grasp. Possibly she could intuit with her fingers what her eyes used to tell her about a person's psyche. Flo's intensity was uncontainable. Her smile was a beacon, her grip was a vise. Her pattern of speech was like a series of small explosions. This was not a woman who was going to let us gracefully glide through psychiatric nursing without getting our fingers sticky.

We sat in the classroom arranged lecture style, waiting for Mrs. Davidson to descend upon us. She entered the room, and her presence filled up every cubic inch of space available to her. She beamed her smile, shook her curly head and said "No, you are not going to sit like this." Our last bit of control was taken away. We were forced to sit in a circle giving Flo Davidson full frontal access to each of us. Now we were to go around the room introducing ourselves to her, and describing any previous psychiatric experience we may have had.

It can be a decided advantage to keep past experience to yourself. On the other hand, an instructor may feel a sense of kindred spirit towards a student whose experience lies in their area of expertise. Watching Evelyn, I have noticed that she always chooses to play dumb, never volunteering any information.

I debated my decision as Flo worked her way around to me. I had pretty much decided to take Evelyn's lead and play dumb, when Flo fixed her eyes on me. I find it impossible to lie to intelligent people who appear to have an innate sense of the truth. I spilled my guts to Flo. "I am a U.S.C. graduate with a major in psych and one year of graduate work in sociology. I plan to go into psychiatric nursing when I graduate." Flo smiled, thoroughly pleased.

Flo told us we must get involved, we must think, we must learn to conceptualize. This was a very vague term as Flo used it. It meant to form a concept or an idea, a theory. Dim-witted people drove her nuts. I understand; they are a struggle for me, too. But Flo took lack of intelligence personally. It was as if she felt all God's creatures were gifted the same, and some were just too lazy to use the stuff between their ears. Students, who couldn't follow her abstract thinking, were her bane. She would get right up in the student's face and demand, "You must learn to conceptualize!" This intimidated the hell out of her students, since they had no idea what she was talking about.

I could usually figure out what Flo was looking for. It took a series of circuitous thoughts to follow her track, but if I hung in there I could sort out the answers to the puzzles she presented. This and my ability to role play (I am especially good at crazy people) endeared me to Flo. I was going to be perfect in psychiatry. I would have no problem getting an "A" in this course.

Conceptualizing and role playing for Flo were relatively easy classroom gymnastics. The hard stuff was waiting for me on the unit. What was it going to be like dealing with crazy people? We weren't calling patients crazy in the classroom. They were manic depressive, schizophrenic, suicidal, depressed, compulsive, phobic, anything but crazy. The one word lurking in our minds, behind all the rhetoric, was crazy.

There was only one psych unit I wanted to be on, 6A. I had heard all about this unit from others who had the class before me. All of the other units were for adults. Adult psych patients didn't hold much allure for me. They were mostly described as chronic, which sounded pretty depressing. 6A was the adolescent crisis unit; the age range ran from fourteen to seventeen. When a patient turned eighteen they were transferred to an adult unit.

I had heard great stories about the head doctor on 6A, Dr. Susan Blade. They told me her mind worked like an automatic weapon, firing off questions, bang, bang, bang. She presided over "group" several mornings a week. She was a woman with a mind and a mouth to be wary of. I really wanted to see her run these group sessions. I knew it was where I was supposed to be. My mind could not entertain any possible alternative.

When the assignments were posted everyone crowded around the bulletin board to see what they had gotten. Michael was standing in front of me, his shoulder blocking my view. He groaned and turned around snarling, "I can't believe it, you always get the best assignment." He moved off before I could find my name on the list. There it was, the reason Michael had been groaning, I was on 6A, and so was Sam. This was great, I was in. I wouldn't have to find someone to change with me, explaining why I must have 6A, and how they probably wouldn't like it anyway.

Four of us had been assigned to 6A. Intimidated and quiet, we followed Flo into the elevator and up to the unit. The elevator doors opened onto a corridor, 6A to the right, 6B to the left. We stood facing a locked heavy metal door with a small window in it. We waited while Flo rang the bell for someone to let us in.

One wants to appear professional, relaxed, and confidant, when entering a psychiatric unit. So we tried to be discrete as the four of us craned our necks and stepped on each other's toes attempting to see in the small window. A heavy-set woman in blue jeans took her time ambling down the hall. There was the sound of keys jangling, a lock turning and then the heavy door swung open. Flo was friendly and happy, totally at home. She clackity-clacked down the hall in her high heels, eager to announce her presence.

It's hard to feel confident and professional following behind a parade like Flo. The chances of blending in unnoticed are absolutely blown. There was no time to quietly observe. We were referred to as baby chicks, neophytes, and little lambs, ready to be initiated. Feeling self-conscious and foolish, we were introduced to some of the nursing staff, and to Annie Sherman, the head nurse. Mrs. Sherman is a four foot eleven ball of energy. She handled the introductions in a brusque, businesslike manner. We were told morning group would be starting in ten minutes, we might want to grab a seat.

Group was to take place in the day room. For some reason psychiatric hospitals call their main lounge area a day room. 6A was "L" shaped, with two long wings of bedrooms forming the legs of the "L". The boys slept in the back section, while the girls slept in the hall that led to the front door. Where the two wings met there was a large lounge, and this was the day room. The nursing station, with Mrs. Sherman's office, was around the corner from the lounge. It had a large window along the back wall that looked out into the day room. Two other sides of the office were also glass, providing a pretty good view of the unit.

Sam and I exchanged glances of nervous anticipation as we left the office and headed for the day room. We were looking around at the kids. Many were normal looking teenagers. A couple were in hospital pajamas; the rest wore their regular clothes. Several of the girls wore make-up and had spent time doing their hair. At first glance the place didn't seem too different from a local high school. As we looked around and I began to focus on individuals, I could see the variation.

Some kids looked absolutely normal. They were alert, dressed like they were ready for school, smart-mouthing around, and playing with each other. Others were distracted, as if they were somewhere else. Their grooming was poor, their attention span was zero. A few of the patients were moving in slow motion. They looked confused and lethargic. I figured these must be the crazy ones. I felt like I was visiting the zoo, and there were no bars between myself and the animals.

I think other people must have felt similarly when first coming to work on a psych unit, but it is unacceptable to say so. I pretended "Hey, this is fine, nice kids." Two of the other nursing students, girls in their early twenties, sat down and started to chat with some of the kids on the unit. I wasn't ready to do that. Some of these kids looked real sick to me, and I was at a loss for where to begin.

You can't hang back looking stiff on a unit of teenagers; they won't stand on politeness and give you some time to acclimate. These kids are locked up on a sterile-looking unit, with very little to entertain them beyond a TV and some games. They are looking for something new and intriguing to catch their eye. New student nurses are perfect to relieve the regular routine of the day. We were toys to be played with, prodded, and probed. We didn't have to make conversation, the kids were ready to grill us and check us out from the moment we appeared.

I sat down on a small three person couch near the window. There was a boy sitting in a chair on my right. He was watching me carefully, studying me. I looked at him and smiled. I wanted to be a psychosocial nurse, open and receptive to this young man. I also got a bit caught up in competitiveness. This is an extremely stupid thing to do. Knee-jerk, competitive behavior tends to push clear, rational thought aside. I hate competition, but at the same time I can get blindly sucked into competitive behavior eradicating all rational thought.

There were those other cute young student nurses, carelessly chatting away with crazy kids. I'll be dammed if I can't perform as well as they can. I smiled more warmly to the boy next to me and said hello. I took a better look at him. He looked to be a good-sized sixteen year-old. He had kind of a weird look in his eye, but otherwise he seemed fairly normal. He told me to come closer as he leaned toward me. I now took a second look and realized he was secured to the chair by a belt around his waist, and leather cuffs on each wrist.

I didn't want to look like I was intimidated because a patient needed a little physical restraining. So when the boy repeated, "come here," I figured he wanted to tell me something. I was a psychiatric nurse, I was all ears. I slid my way over closer, ready to hear his innermost feelings.

Instantly, he grabbed my wrist. I hadn't realized he could reach that far. With unbelievable power, the kid held onto me like a vise. "Shit", I thought, "now what do I do, scream for help and look like an idiot?" The answer is, of course you scream for help, immediately. Competitor to the end, I hadn't regained my senses. I was still trying to maintain some modicum of cool. I had hesitated too long, thinking maybe I could talk him out of this behavior. He gave my wrist a hard twist, taking me right to my knees.

I found my self on the floor of the day room, scrambling to get my legs under me. My wrist was fixed at an intensely painful angle. I was still not yelling for help. I was still thinking, "I can get out of this, my dignity can be saved. Thank God I am wearing pants!" He only had a hold of my wrist. I couldn't believe how totally incapacitated I was. I flailed on the ground at his feet. I began to wonder if I was going to die down there. But never could I do something so uncool as to yell, "Get this fucker off of me!"

Psychiatric nursing attendants love new medical and nursing students. We were better than the Three Stooges, Laurel and Hardy all rolled together. Mr. Grant, one of the attendants, had allowed me to twist in my fate for as long as his sense of decency would let him. If it had been up to his sense of humor I might have died there. Fortunately, Grant is a very decent man. His strong, bulky form towered over me. His tone was patronizing, barely controlling his laughter, as he told the boy, "Let her go Carl". And that was all it took, I was a free woman.

With the tiny ounce of dignity I had left, I gracelessly pulled myself up from the floor. I rose to my feet as a slightly smarter woman. I had learned some important lessons for surviving on 6A. Number One: Do not assume a situation can not get worse, ever! Number Two: Attendants have the power to save your life, or not, depending on their mood. These are not people to take lightly. Number Three: Screaming and looking like a fool is better than getting hurt, even if you end up the butt of everyone's jokes for the next ten months.

I was shaken and humiliated by my first encounter on psych. I was also determined to hang in there and stay together. I camouflaged my emotions to the best of my ability. I made heroic attempts to quiet my breathing and control my shakes. Mr. Grant politely asked if I was OK. I lied, "I'm fine, no problem, he just took me by surprise." Mr. Grant was a dear, he didn't even laugh in my face. He just said "Right." I walked with all the dignity I could find, to a seat near the back of the room.

The patients were beginning to arrange themselves for morning group. One side of the day room had a horseshoe arrangement of couches and chairs for convenient TV. watching. This is where I had been sitting earlier next to the "stationary chair." They had a heavy arm chair bolted to the ground. They could place a patient there if he or she needed to be restrained and the staff wanted them in the day room. The kids began to jockey for position and take their places forming a circle. My pal Carl was still well secured to the stationary chair.

One of the boys carried two chairs over and placed them in front of the TV. These were for Dr. Susan Blade, the head of 6A, and her second in command, Dr. Dilan Davis. Interns, residents, and medical students who were currently assigned to 6A, took seats or perched themselves around the other end of the room to observe. Nursing staff and attendants came and went as they liked. Annie Sherman frequently came in and stood by the door, watching the proceedings.

On my first few visits it was all a mystery to me, how everything came about, who was where, and why. I would eventually join this group. 6A was going to become my territory, and I would be at home there, just like the rest of the staff. But on my first day I sat curious and excited, waiting for group to begin. I wondered what SHE would be like.

Susan Blade takes the floor the moment she enters a room. I was shocked by her appearance, and at the same time it made perfect sense. I was expecting some sort of serious psychiatric doctor who knows what I thought that would be. I wasn't expecting Joan Rivers in silk and wool, gold and diamonds, a short-haired blond with freckles who would flop into a chair and pick at her long, two-toned manicured nails. Susan could fuss with her nails, admire her own lovely silk blouse, then look up and fire off the most intensely personal questions I had ever heard.

The effect was mesmerizing. I fell into immediate infatuation and girl-love. Girl-love is the way I felt about my camp counselor named Susie, who knew more than anybody in the world about animals, trees, and Winnie The Pooh. Infatuation with an admirable woman, wishing you could spend an evening together in front of the fire, drinking wine, eating ice cream and pop corn, and talking all night, is what girl-love is all about. I get lots of crushes on women who I think are wonderful and I wish I could know. Writers are some of my favorites. I want to spend a day riding horses with Rita Mae Brown, and I want to lunch with Maya Angelou. I have crushes on Whoopie Goldberg and Lily Tomlin.

I sat in the day room a bundle of emotions and excitement as I intently followed the progress of this morning's group. Susan's focus bounced pinball style from one patient to the next. She began with the alert kids. Some were obviously eager to talk. They wanted to tell her everything about themselves, and about everyone else on the unit, too.

Watching the group carefully, I began to get a better understanding of the patient population on 6A. The crazy kids were in the minority, a small handful somewhere between three to five. There were a couple who were dusted on P.C.P., known as angel dust, it was the children's drug of the day. The rest appeared to be pretty normal teenagers, coping with major stress at home, school, or wherever. I learned this through Susan's questioning. For the sake of the new patients and student nurses, she asked the kids how they came to be on the unit. The reason for admission for the majority of patients was a suicide attempt.

This was shocking when I first came face to face with it. There was no visible signs that marked these kids as suicidal. Some were so well packaged that they could be running for president of their high school. One girl was a senior class president. Other kids, I could look at them, and see the pain. These kids were slovenly and depressed or anxious. Several looked flat of affect or haunted. I had not realized how much danger from their own hand a child like this was in.

I didn't understand, on that first day, that a major source of the variety in the appearance of patients was due to the stages they go through while on the unit. The stages were especially prominent in the kids who weren't crazy. They would arrive looking wild, disheveled, hollow-eyed, exhausted, and frightened. The nursing staff took control first. A new patient was showered, and put in pajamas. Their belongings were temporarily confiscated. If the child was alert enough they would be interviewed and assessed by an R.N. If not, they would be put to bed in the hall outside the nursing office, where everyone could keep an eye on them.

An indication of how exhausted a new patient might be is that they could sleep in the hallway, right in the middle of all the hustle and bustle. The hospital beds were on wheels and were moved into the hallway whenever the staff thought there was a need. All new patients spent their first night in the hall, right in front of the nurses. Patients who admitted to feeling like killing themselves, or who acted suicidal, had their beds moved into the hall also. On a morning after a bad night with several new patients, or kids who were looking suicidal, the hall contained a train of white beds.

New patients were kept in hospital pajamas until the staff had enough time to assess them and decide they were stable enough to have their street clothes back. Some kids made it into street clothes the day they were admitted; others took longer. After working on 6A for a while, I could watch the transformation of kids as they stayed there. For many patients the fear and confusion would slowly disappear from their eyes. The drugs would clear from their systems, and a wild-looking child would metamorphose into a pretty normal kid with some serious problems.

The normal kids with serious problems made up about seventy percent of the unit's population, and they did most of the talking in group. They would give the staff tremendous amounts of information. The kids wanted to "get well", to conquer their depression and fears, or to gain independence from craziness at home that they couldn't change. The normal kids were even more pushy about wanting other kids to get well, and to "stop acting crazy." So they would tell you everything that went on; who was making sense, and who wasn't.

If Susan wanted to know how a silent, sulking child was doing, she would ask the group. "How has Mary been, is she making any sense to anybody, or is she still talking crazy?" Frequently she would address her question to the most lucid patient in the group. The kids would tell her what they had seen. They would be frustrated and disappointed if Mary was still acting crazy, or excited and encouraging if she had begun to speak even a word or two of sane stuff.

I believe there is such a thing as true mental illness, and I think much of it is biochemical in nature. About ten percent or so of the kids on 6A ten years ago were clinically labeled mentally ill. There was variety in the types of illness we saw and the effectiveness of treatment. Life on 6A today is very different from what I experienced ten years ago. Changes have take place over the last decade in social patterns, in diagnosis and treatment, and especially in the laws concerning mental patients.

Depression and mania caused by biochemical imbalances were treated fairly effectively. There were moments of tremendous joy following weeks of the entire unit working with a patient when on their last morning in group we said good-bye and good luck to a healthy, confident teenager. There were sorrowful moments, such as watching the parents of a young schizophrenic, talking quietly, holding their child's hand, sitting beside the bed of a child they had probably lost forever to the deep, intractable pain tunnels of schizophrenia.

The last twenty percent of the patients on 6A fell somewhere between troubled and ill. Many of these were drug users. Angel dust was cheap and evil stuff. Of all the types of drug use I have seen, P.C.P. is still the worst stuff out there. Mind bending craziness, a nihilistic power and paranoia and uncontainable insanity is what this shit creates. Kids who smoked it would arrive on the unit in four- and five-point restraints, leather cuffs and belts at the wrists and ankles for four-point, or also at the torso for five-point. The oblivion to pain and the sheer physical power is unbelievable unless you have seen it.

I gained new respect for the L.A.P.D. out there dealing with these people. The fact that they brought any of them in alive was amazing to me. I saw a fifteen-year-old boy throw a hospital bed against the wall repeatedly for an hour, with just the strength of his head and neck muscles; everything else was tied down. Many of these kids would arrive downstairs in the emergency room with the probes of an electric tasar gun, used by the police to subdue them, still attached. I figure the tasar gun has saved the lives of a number of kids on P.C.P.; the only other choice would be to shoot them.

Patients on drugs were given medication to help clear the drugs out of their systems. They were kept in restraints until they were sane enough to be let out. It might take six male attendants to shower one small boy on P.C.P. Usually within twelve to forty-eight hours the child was able to be up and about unrestrained. The meanness would subside, but the crazy, confused thinking took much longer. What was left to the staff was to watch and wait. Most kids would finally clear and begin to think in rational patterns once again.

A few kids never do clear. The drug-induced craziness just won't abate. It is a different kind of craziness than in a mind that is escaping psychic pain. Drug craziness looks more like the wiring in the brain got fried, leaving glassy eyed confusion. 6A is a crisis unit designed for short-term stays. Originally kids stayed about two weeks, but by the time I was there the average stay was four to six weeks. When two months would go by and a kid wouldn't clear up from the drugs, all that was left was a long-term transfer to the state mental hospital.

All of this was discussed in group, who is sick, who has problems, and who is stoned out of their mind. It is not always easy to tell who is who in these situations. Susan would occasionally ask a patient to go around the room and tell her which patients were sick and which had problems. She would ask them to pick out the sickest one in the group. This was important because it helped everyone to look at reality and adjust their expectations. In a world that specializes in deceit and euphemisms, "you aren't crazy, you have problems," or "you are right, you are sick," can be tremendously reassuring things to hear.

The kids were not the only ones trying to sort things out. The staff would constantly debate and assess, is this kid crazy, or is this kid acting out in response to a problem at home? Is this biochemical depression, or is this depression due to some truly sad events? Every patient on the unit was a puzzle to be sorted out, explored and treasured.

The surprising thing to me was how beloved the kids were. The most obnoxious of them would worm their way into some staff member's heart, some quirky little behavior would touch someone's fancy, and the staff member would be won over. This was not a staff who's motto was to "love all the sick little children back to health." There were some real tough folks on this staff, and they were not here to mess around. They were street smart, and life smart. They didn't buy a lot of crap.

The phenomenon of emotionally adopting a child was well recognized on the unit. Every kid appealed to someone. Real charmers who tried hard were no problem, everybody liked them. But others were unexplainable chemistry. Some terrible, hyperactive little liar, who was "crazy as a shithouse rat," would just tickle Mrs. Sherman with his incessant antics. He would become her "son." She was someone who would care for him no matter how horrid he behaved.

Annie is a smart woman. I noticed that her "sons" and "daughters" were always the demanding, hyperactive little ones. They were the kids most likely to drive the rest of her nursing staff to the end of their rope. Being a mother or a father was a dubious honor. Sometimes it was bestowed, "Mr. Grant, your son needs to learn some manners." Sometimes it was claimed, "Don't you talk about my daughter that way." Frequently one regretted the familial relationship, just as biological parents do.

Nevertheless the bonds were there, and they were strong. Teenagers did not pass through 6A unattached. They would arouse feelings in the staff of frustration, anger, pain, joy, delight, and pride. The patients could not remain aloof from each other any more than they could from the staff. They aroused the same complex array of feelings in one another. There was no pretense of objective thinking on the unit. There was always someone to champion a patient's cause, no matter how big a pill they were. I spent a total of about eighteen months on 6A, mostly as a nurse after I graduated. I had my own share of sons and daughters. These are the ones I don't forget. They will always stay with me. I will always carry the torch and hope for them. One always hopes their child will make it.

I began my psychiatric rotation assuming the nurses took care of the patients, the doctors handled the therapy, and the nursing attendants helped the nurses. I pictured a hierarchy, doctors, nurses, and attendants. In real life the only reliable evidence of a hierarchy rested in the pay scale. By the second day on the unit the lines of who did what were beginning to blur for me. By the second week I began to realize the staffing of 6A was a complex social structure, and I was only seeing the surface of it.

I got a better glimpse into the internal workings of the unit in the staff meetings that took place after group. This is when Susan held rounds each morning. Annie told the nursing students they were free to go to rounds if they liked. "If they liked" - there was no where else I wanted to be. As a student nurse I was mostly a silent observer. I realized this group was a complicated, well defined network. It was best not to interject until I was more sure of the footing. I sat on a countertop and watched while the room filled up with people. The room began filling with a potpourri of personalities. During the next few weeks I put names together with job titles and unofficial ranking on the unit.

It quickly became apparent to me that position on the 6A totem pole was determined by how much value Susan Blade placed upon your opinion. In some ways it was the cleanest form of government. If your comments were consistently accurate, insightful, and useful, you were ranked fairly high. If you could manage to be bright, quick and funny too, you were assured a spot at the top. If your thoughts tended to be mundane, simplistic, or flowed at too slow of a rate, your ranking on Susan's pole was very low.

There were some inherent problems in this system. Occasionally, an insightful thought could be easily overlooked, if it was spouted by someone who was not recognized as bright. Not only did the thoughts determine the value of the source, but the source also determined the value of the thoughts. This system's only chance is if you have a tremendously impartial judge sitting above it all, evaluating each thought on its own merit.

Susan, however, was only human. She had her pets and favorites. If your mind ran at the normal clip, if you didn't have a bent for the sardonic, then your only hope was to become Susan's sycophant. Otherwise, you were doomed to being a second rate citizen on 6A. Since the treatment aspect of the unit worked by compiling input, distilling it, and evaluating the findings to form a plan of action, your purpose on the unit was greatly neutralized if your opinion wasn't valued.

One day of watching morning rounds was enough for me to understand this. A shy therapist gave an opinion, and it laid there on the floor like an accident. The social worker tossed off a snide comment, and received a round of kudos for her insight. This lesson was not lost on me. I studied the group, and their reactions. I watched to see what they wanted.

They wanted to be entertained, and the one you had to entertain most was Susan. These people were not looking for silly jokes or empty amusements. They were extremely serious about their work. They were also jaded and impatient. Their track history for getting kids out of the mire and on their feet was very good. Their minds were seeking insights, solutions and alternative paths that might work. This is what entertained them. If you couldn't be creative, you had damned well better be funny, because wit was the only the only other saving grace.

I paid close attention to these dynamics while I kept my mouth shut. Susan must have viewed this as a sign of my intelligence. By the time I had finished my eight weeks rotation on psych, I was considered 6A property. I was recruited and claimed as their own. I was given a good position on the totem pole. It was assumed I would join the elite, and I was thrilled. They were exactly the group I had wanted. My job as a graduate nurse was secured. I had found my niche in nursing.

This is not unusual in a place like County. Head nurses watch the County students coming through with a hunter's eye. They look for the exceptional students and quickly offer them positions upon graduation. Different units need different skills. Each staff has its unique temperament; personalities that will blend well with the group are highly prized. Hard workers will be told frequently throughout their career as a student that they will be welcomed back as an R.N., if they choose. Occasionally, if a head nurse feels strongly, the statement is made more dramatically. With the reaction I received on 6A I felt a bit like a gold mine. I was delighted to be so highly prized, but I was also a little wary of people staking out a claim on me.

The biggest claim made on me was by Annie Sherman. The head nurses are always a little intimidating because they are the ones you ultimately have to please. Annie had a quick, fiery mind. She didn't stand back and look at things intellectually. She got down and dirty with the staff and the patients. If the kids needed a big dose of mean mother, she would storm into the dayroom, roaring like a lion from hell. She would also carefully hold any bruised heart that needed it. This is what made her "hellcat" act so effective.

When Annie's dander was up, Grant and the other men would stick on her tail. When she was inflamed, Mrs. Sherman would forget she was five feet tall. She would get right up in the face of anybody who pissed her off. The men were ready to save her life in case some kid should finally let her have it. But Annie never noticed the men behind her. She said her piece, turned her back on the lambasted kid, and walked away.

In the beginning Annie's act frightened me. I saw the fire before I got a chance to see the softness. I figured this lady could eat me for breakfast; so I toed the mark. I am a very diligent employee; for Annie, I was nearly compulsive. It wasn't tough, because the work was exciting and important. Admiration is contagious. Annie was delighted with me. I was dubbed her "daughter", and her best friend's "niece". The week I came to work on 6A as an R.N., the adoption was completed.

Chapter Twenty-Two

The Girls Go Traveling

It was spring break and we were coming into the home stretch of nursing school. It seemed to me like the time was right for a major International Coffee moment. What we needed was a "girl trip." We needed a cheap trip, because none of us had much money. I convinced Evelyn and Susan that Pebble Beach was the perfect destination because my parents have a vacation home there. I was talking three days, no hotel costs, a private room for each of us so we wouldn't get too crazy with one another, and the most beautiful location on the face of the planet.

I was nervous about taking my friends to the Monterey Peninsula. It is my favorite place on earth. I wasn't sure they would appreciate it and love it appropriately. I wasn't sure how Evelyn would feel hanging out in an all-white preserve. I figured she would do better than Susan, who's political beliefs assume that all white people with money probably got it by stealing babies from blind mothers, and then selling them to their friends as cheap domestic labor.

I was afraid my friends wouldn't feel the thunder as the waves pounded the rocks. They might not sense Mother Earth's hand on their shoulders, whispering in their ears, as they watched a newborn fawn in the forest. Here the forest joins the sea in an explosion of foam and salt. The shore is wild and rocky. The waves can sweep you in, never to release you. There is power in the air, strength in the trees. I couldn't say to my friends, "Look, I want to show you a part of my soul." Normal people don't talk like that. I would have scared them to death. I was going to hold my most cherished place on Earth in my hands and carefully spread them open for my friends to see. But, the bribe I used to get them there was to say it would be cheap. I packed my friends in my V.W., and we took off.

The trip was tricky to begin with because both Evelyn and Susan smoke. These women love their cigarettes. They each smoked their own brand and they were not interchangeable. Cigarette smoke makes my nose burn and drives my allergies nuts. I don't harass my friends who smoke, but when it comes to my home and my car there is no smoking allowed.

When smokers are around my home they step outside to light up, and I usually keep them company. When the three of us hung out at the dorms, smoking went on in Evelyn or Susan's rooms. We would stay in my room until someone needed a cig, and then we would move to their place. This is not possible when three people are stuck in a V.W. for six hours.

There had to be compromise. We would never make it if we had to stop every fifteen minutes for a smoke. I made a decision, "OK, you guys can smoke, if you keep all the windows rolled down." Susan bitched about her hair blowing, and I responded by telling her not to leave any ashes in my car. The radio was cranked up blaring Country and Western tunes. Susan was ready to barf from the music, but she was pacified by having received permission to puff. Evelyn was a happy cat. She sat in the front seat singing along with me to the radio, and puffing away with Susan.

We cruised on and on, finally stopping at Anderson's Split Pea place for lunch. We made it up to Pebble Beach, and nosed our way down my parents' steep drive just as darkness was settling in. I jumped out of the car, filled my nose with cold forest air, and beamed like a lighthouse. Peace and joy filled my heart. I was home again. I looked around to see my friends tentatively stepping out of the car. Susan looked up at the sky, as if she didn't trust it, "It sure is dark out here." Evelyn stood close to Susan, trying to discern shapes in the evening forest. She repeated Susan's lament, "It sure is dark out here."

I was slow to catch on. "Yeah, isn't it great? The dark nights are the best part, the stars shine so bright." My friends looked at me with doubt. I decided it was better to move them inside quickly, so I reached behind the flower pot and fished out the key. Rather than being reassured of the safety of a neighborhood where one can leave a key in an obvious place, Evelyn and Susan looked horrified. I had brought them to somewhere primitive. I was sure their anxieties would be soothed when they saw the inside of the house.

People who have heard of Pebble Beach, or even driven the Seventeen Mile scenic drive, usually think all of the homes there are mansions. There are mansions, and they are building even more on a daily basis. But there are also moderate family homes that line the winding internal streets of the Seventeen Mile Drive. This is the sort of house my parents have, cozy, homey, not at all palatial. The house is not the least bit primitive; it is comforting and welcoming.

Susan and Evelyn seemed reassured once they got inside and locked the doors. I built a big fire, and everyone took a room. We had three days ahead of us to enjoy the Monterey Peninsula and experience the out-of-doors. I unpacked my clothes and returned to the living room to enjoy the fire. I found my friends huddled together on the deck having a cigarette, staying as close to the porch light as possible. I figured it was time to open a bottle of wine.

I had never given any thought to the idea that my two city friends might not be charmed by the woods. Susan's concept of the beach was the Marina in Long Beach. She had pictures of lying out in a bikini on warm sand, gently lapped by two-inch waves, where one is never far from a place to sit and have a cold beer, smoke a cig and watch the people go by. She did not find a rocky coast, thundering waves, and a cold breeze invigorating. She figured the three of us would freeze our tits off lying out on a beach like this, and none of us could afford to lose any inches.

Evelyn could hang with things a little better. She wasn't as prone to bitch right up as Susan was. But I knew she wasn't charmed. Had I been thinking clearly, I would have realized what to do in a case like this. Go shopping! Carmel By the Sea is minutes away, and loaded with shops so cute they could kill you. City girls can always make themselves at home in places that take Visa and Mastercard. I should have saved the day and hustled my buds to the shops, the taverns, and the people. I didn't because that wasn't what I really wanted to show them. I was determined for them to know and love "my peninsula."

The first day we drove around, showing my friends the majesty of the peninsula. The best part for them may have been that every time we stopped to get out and look at something, they could have a smoke. The three of us could have a good time almost anywhere, laughing and talking, so we weren't too miserable, but it just wasn't magic. I decided day two should be special. We would go hiking, or really just for a long walk. All the signals were there for me that this was not a great idea, but I pushed forward.

I began by explaining how nice it would be, "We could just walk down the hill to the beach, about an hour round trip, no big deal. One hour, anybody can walk one hour, right?" For some reason my friends went along with me. I had become the troop leader for three days. It was a burden I quickly came to loathe. The walk down to the beach was nice, a fifteen to twenty minute downhill stroll. We walked through streets lined with oaks and pine trees. We passed deer, squirrels, and blue jays.

We walked along the ocean, we peered through the telescopes at Bird and Seal Rock. We were having a pretty good time. For the return trip I thought, let's do something more interesting than the road. Let's go back through the marsh and forest. I thought this was a great idea. No, there wasn't a path or trail, but how lost can you get, it is a relatively small strip of forest. Off the road, down a low grassy slope, I led our trio to a small, pristine marsh. The cat tails were shoulder high and the red-winged black birds were flaring their color in the sun. We could walk up the marsh along the tiny river into the forest.

I thought this was great. We could pretend we were explorers. Evelyn and Susan thought their shoes were getting very muddy. Neither took this well; you should never mess with some women's shoes. Muddy shoes are bad, but we were almost in the forest, where, I assured them, it would be dryer. I was a thoughtful guide. I pointed out the different wild life, and the poison oak. I told them "Don't touch the poison oak, it will give you a bad rash."

Being surrounded by poisonous plants was too much to bear that required a cigarette break. My friends huddled together in that eternal battle of smoker against nature trying to light a match. Being a non-smoker, I have never been in that huddle to find out what goes on. Their heads were pressed close together, they talked a lot, cussed a lot, and used up a book of matches. Suddenly they emerged looking triumphant and smug, cigarettes glowing in both of their hands. They sat on a log, side by side, to enjoy this bonding moment, while I noodled around in the plants.

A spew of obscenities came blasting out of Susan's mouth as she jumped, kicked, and screamed. Evelyn was panicking, smacking her body everywhere. "Bugs, the God-damn log has bugs." The plants are poisonous, the ground is muddy, and the trees have bugs. Our hike was beginning to degrade. I said "OK, lets just hike through this little patch of forest up to the road, we can stay on the paved street from there." My friends agreed that at the top of this little hill, we would take the road.

I don't know what happened, the road should have been there, I was sure of it. But it wasn't, and they were not happy. I had two city girls just a little lost in the woods, running low on matches, with mud on their nice shoes. No one felt the need to pretend any longer that they were having fun. I had better get them to civilization, which meant cigarettes, matches, beer, and clean feet, soon. I told them not to panic, it was a very tiny patch of woods, we couldn't be too lost.

The tiny patch of woods decided not to release us for another hour. It was then another thirty-five minutes walk by road back to the house. My pals immediately purged their bodies of all residue of the outdoors. They grabbed a couple of beers, and headed to the deck for a cig. I left them alone until they had a chance to sate all their civilized needs. Warmed by the beer and the smoke, they took me back into their good graces. I promised no more off-path trekking.

We spent our last day indulging ourselves with food, wine, cards and gossip. We talked about my romance with Jeff - where would it go, did I want to get married, did we want to have kids. Jeff and I had an argument right before the trip. I have no idea now what it was about. I do remember the lousy feeling of going out of town when things between us were unsettled. I was worried about what I would come home to. I didn't want to tell Susan and Evelyn that I wasn't sure where our relationship was going.

We rolled into County at seven p.m., just in time to catch the worst meal of the week, mystery pizza. We parted in the elevator, Susan and I getting off on the seventh floor, Evelyn going on up to the ninth. We would meet in fifteen minutes at Susan's to go to dinner. It was a pretty good sign that our friendship had survived the trip.

I found a package sitting on my desk, a large basket full of eggs and candy. I had forgotten today was Easter. Jeff had bribed someone official to break into my room and leave the gift. I untied the bow and folded back the red cellophane wrapping. In the center of the jelly beans and marshmallow egg was a delicate egg shell. It had been blown out, cleaned, and hand painted. I saw my face in profile, wearing my blue quilted cap, a rainbow trailing behind my head. He had left a card depicting one heart speaking to another, and the meaning of friendship. I am still learning the meaning of friendship and loving. They evolve and present themselves anew to me, as I live and watch and change.

Chapter Twenty-Three

Macho Nursing

All the fun rotations were finished. Peds, Psych, and Obstetrics were now behind me. What was left was the serious stuff. I had been dreading the real nursing, Advanced Medical\Surgical Nursing 202 and 203. This was my senior rotation, with one instructor left between myself and graduation. Actually, there were three instructors left because our whole class was back together again for our final term. Our large lecture class would be taught by Mary and Marie Mason.

It was almost like having two instructors for lecture, because Mary and Marie were identical twins, somewhere in their late twenties or early thirties. The women were still identical - their hair, clothes, make-up, everything. I never knew who I was talking to and this unsettled me. Some people said they could tell them apart because one was prettier than the other. For me, this was splitting hairs. There is a picture of each of them in our annual. It looks like a the same picture was printed twice. There was something spooky about two grown women who chose to maintain a joint identity. If they came to County on their days off, they would wear matching play clothes.

The mystique of the Clones, as they came to be known, was intensified by their being incredibly tough instructors. Terrifying twins, teaching the toughest class in nursing school. The rumors spread, and students broke out in sweats as they walked by. I was one of those sweating. When we were broken up into clinical groups for 202 and 203, I prayed not to be given one of the Clones as my small group instructor. The Gods perpetrated one last act of kindness on me in nursing school. I was assigned Gilbert Richardson as my final clinical instructor.

The last term is called 202 and 203 because it is broken up into two sections. The first section focused on our nursing skills. The second section was team leading to hone our leadership skills. We were assigned to the most difficult units in the hospital, the places with the heaviest work loads like the burn unit and oncology. Gilbert supervised his students on two units, neurosurgery and infected orthopedics. We would spend six weeks on each unit. We were allowed to choose which of these two we wanted to work on for our final rotation in team leading.

Gilbert was a middle-sized, stocky man, with playful blue eyes. He had a British accent, charm, and a sense of humor. He was a military-trained nurse and very competent. I had labeled the type of nursing we were about to undertake as Macho Nursing. The men thrived on it. Tubes, bed sores, coma cases, suction pumps, massive wounds, really gruesome stuff. Macho nurses eat it up. They love to tell you over dinner exactly how horrible their unit is. I had heard these stories in the cafeteria for a year and a half now. My sense of what made it all so macho was the nurses' ability to emotionally distance themselves from the humanity of their patients. Being tough was a necessity for getting a tough job done.

Throughout school I had not shown any great talent for distancing myself from patients. I was afraid 202 and 203 might just wipe me out. Gilbert Richardson's job was to put me to the test; could I handle it? Supposedly, we knew the basics of nursing. Now was the time to sort us out, to find out how good we really were. Many nursing schools are much cleaner, much more theoretical. It doesn't get this dirty. I instinctively knew County would be about the hardest. I knew classes like 202 and 203 were out there waiting for me. They were some of the monsters I had to face. They had something to do with why I chose County.

My first six weeks under Gilbert's supervision were spent on infected orthopedics, also known as the "pus ward." This was a closed unit, meaning if any staff member was sick the absence was covered by others who worked on the unit. The staff came in on their days off or worked extra shifts to prevent other hospital nurses, unfamiliar with the unit, from being floated there to work. The work on infected ortho required special attention and thought. The patients all had problems involving their bones; usually they were broken. They also had infected wounds to compound their problems.

Patients on this unit were here for long stays. Almost every patient was on intravenous antibiotics, generally receiving a four-week course. There were patients in isolation with penicillin-resistant infections. Wounds ranged from human bites, generally on the knuckle area, and received in a bar room, to shredded limbs from motor cycle accidents. I felt strongly about two things after working infected ortho. Never hit someone in the mouth, and asphalt does terrible things to a body when contacted at high speeds.

The head nurse was Cheryl South, an average size woman with a sturdy build, and dark hair. Cheryl was in her late twenties, or early thirties. She commanded and received great respect and loyalty from her staff. The year after I graduated Cheryl South and Annie Sherman were each nominated by their staff for Nurse of the Year at County, and both made it into the finals. Our first day on the unit Cheryl showed up immaculately groomed from head to toe in crisp white, including her County graduate's nursing cap.

Working nurses rarely wear their caps (of course the Clones always did) but normally this archaic piece of uniform is just too impractical. Cheryl announced she had decided to wear her cap because she thought it might command more respect than she had been getting lately. There was a spark in her eye as she said this. Many patients stayed on this unit so long they began to feel they owned it. If they didn't own the unit they at least felt they had dibs on Cheryl. Frustrated men, who had been confined to bed far too long for any male ego to tolerate, would vie for Cheryl's attention, making demands.

Suddenly, the only person who could touch some man's dressing change or settle a dispute was Cheryl. A patient might throw a tantrum just to have Cheryl stop her busy routine and stand by their side to lay down the law. She was mother, sister, and sweetheart to the predominantly male unit, all bedridden beyond their patience. Every once in a while Cheryl would toughen up. She would tell the whiners and fussers to shape up, no more crap. The effect of all this professionalism was temporary, but it allowed Cheryl to catch up on her paperwork.

The morning began with Karen, the charge nurse on the night shift, giving her change-of-shift report. Here changes in anyone's status was noted, especially any rise in temperature, a sign of infection. Karen was petite, dark, and sarcastic. She could never just give a straight report. Orthopedics does attract a lot of colorful patients, and their acting out is intensified by their prolonged stays. Karen editorialized her entire way through rounds. Her smart mouth was infamous. There was always a crowd around her as she gave her end-of-shift report.

Toward the end of report we arrived at Olivia's private room. Some patients require private rooms because their infections are so vile you try to prevent contaminating other patients. A few select souls get private rooms because they are so nasty or crazy that it would be unfair to put someone with them. Olivia fell into the latter category. She was a jumper, someone who jumps from high places to do themselves bodily harm. She was an unsuccessful jumper, the type who repeatedly jumps from places high enough to injure, but low enough not to kill.

Olivia usually came to infected ortho from the psych unit where she spent most of her time. She drove almost everyone on the staff nuts except Karen. Olivia frequently saw men in her room. Under the chairs, in the closet, behind the door, these men were waiting to get her, and she couldn't sleep. We had been carefully trained in psych never to enter into a patient's delusion. This is counter-productive. A professional nurse assures the patient that there are no men hiding in the corners, and allows the patient to re-examine their fears. A busy nurse offers the patient sleeping medication. Karen grabbed a broom and beat the hell out of all those men hiding in the corners. Olivia was well entertained, and slept like a baby.

Much too soon for me, nursing rounds were over and I was assigned my patients. Because of the complexity of the care required, we were only given two. My first one had a human bite on his hand and the other had mangled his leg in a motorcycle accident. The first thing I had to do was look up my patients' care plans at the nursing station. There was a detailed description of each patient's wound care. I figured it was best to start small. I went for the guy with the bite.

I had already done a morning check, meeting these men and taking care of their immediate needs, bed pans, clean linens, etc., before looking up my instructions for tackling dressing changes. Mr. John Martin was a strong, young, healthy male, who had abruptly stuck his fist in somebody's mouth. This was a bad move. His hand had become infected and was terribly swollen. The swelling and pus caused enough tissue damage to require surgery and he was now receiving antibiotics intravenously. John had been stuck in County fourteen days now because he had gotten drunk and punched somebody.

I have heard many nurses debate whether they prefer male or female patients. Supposedly females are cleaner, more tolerant of pain, but very demanding. Males, on the other hand, are thought to have fewer expectations and to be less demanding. They are also considered messier, and are much bigger babies. I like working with both; however I do find there are some kernels of truth in the stereotypes.

John Martin had a relatively small wound, about three square inches with one deep puncture, and a very low pain tolerance. I approached John cheerfully, bearing a small sterile bundle. I also had the hydrogen peroxide for irrigating his wound. I did my Mother Merlin routine, setting up a beautiful sterile field. I put on a pair of clean gloves, saving the sterile ones for later. I was all ready, smiling by John's side, the perfect nurse.

It was time to remove the soiled dressing. I really hate this part, not knowing what it's going to look like when I take off the bandage. Before I touched the tape, I cemented my face into a pleasant look. I told my muscles to hold that face no matter what. It's the Charley's Angels version of nursing, smiling sweetly while ripping adhesive from a very hairy arm. A tiny rrrip, and John let out a big "Oww, that hurts". My facial muscles do not have the guerilla warfare training of a newscaster's. I collapsed in a frown and looked at John.

I don't merely loathe causing people pain. I have a nearly pathological aversion to it. With people or animals, I have to work very hard to separate myself from their misery. My dogs think discipline refers to my controlling my anger when they poop on the carpet. If I had children, they would probably end up terrorists. I felt immediately resentful towards John. I wanted to be the painless nurse and here he was yelling as soon as I touched him. If he hadn't slugged somebody, I wouldn't now have to cause him pain.

In truth, it was my fault I was in this situation. I had chosen to go to nursing school, but right now I was angry and regretting it. I still hadn't removed the bandage. My anxiety rose as I imagined the horrors underneath it. Poor John. I was overcome with the double dread of pus and pain. I took my self-anger balled it up nicely and plopped it on John's head. Having securely fixed John as the source of my irritation, it was a little easier to proceed.

I was transformed from one of Chuck's Broads into "the firm nurse." "This will only take a moment, yelling won't help." Rrrrrrip. The bandage was now in my hand. I held onto it while inverting my plastic glove as I took the glove off. The soiled bandage was now safely encased in plastic. I squinted and bent my head closer to take a look at John's hand. He remained quiet, examining me with an untrusting eye.

This was a tiny wound. It had healed over and was now only an inch-and-a-half long. There was still a round puncture needing deeper cleaning. John and I looked into each other's disappointed eyes. "It used to be much bigger," he told me, justifying his pain and anguish. He yelled again when I inserted the long-stem swab into the puncture to clean it out. He groaned as I rinsed the wound out with hydrogen peroxide. We were in a large room with seven other men. Surrounding us were men in traction unable to move and men with smashed limbs in terrible pain. Here John was with his tiny wound, his bottle of antibiotics dripping into his arm, feeling like a fool. Poor John, it's hell to be at the bottom of the sympathy totem pole. I didn't help matters any for him. I am sure I was forever cast in his mind as "The Bitch."

After finishing with John, I took my angel of mercy act over to the nursing station to prepare for my next patient. I think part of the tension that I had vented on John was in anticipation of my next patient. Stephen Mitchell was a friendly twenty-two year old who had nearly destroyed his right leg in a motorcycle accident. I had put off treating him as long as I could. It was now time to go deal with Stephen's leg.

I collected a huge sterile bundle, and a couple of small ones. I grabbed an orange juice out of the refrigerator and drank it, so hopefully I wouldn't faint while I worked. I took a copy of the complicated dressing change directions with me. They were too complex to memorize, and I didn't want to miss anything. I arrived at Stephen's side, and asked, "Well, are you ready?" He said the pain meds had started taking effect and he thought he could handle it now. For the serious dressing changes the nurses tried to time them so the patients would be premedicated.

Stephen's leg was up in traction with a sheet draped tent style over most of it. He didn't like people seeing his leg. I pulled the curtains surrounding his bed, enclosing us in a private world of white. I took a deep breath and gently removed the sheet. It was time to begin. Metal pins for the traction weights were inserted at his hip, knee, and ankle. The bolts projected from his skin to give the ropes and pulleys places to attach. His upper thigh and knee were laced with surgical scars. From the knee to the ankle almost all the flesh was missing from Stephen's leg. His bones were exposed and starting to turn brown like an old skeleton in an anatomy class. Vaseline and gauze were laid over his exposed tendons in an attempt to prevent their drying out. A small portion of flesh remained on his calf. Through this traversed the only arteries, veins, and nerves keeping his foot alive. Stephen's foot remained mostly intact, stranded at the distal end of his exposed bones.

"It looks pretty bad, doesn't it?"

"Yeah," I said, "it looks bad. How's the pain right now?"

"I can handle it. I'm gonna keep my leg. They're gonna save it."

"God, that's amazing, that's wonderful. I can't believe what they are able to do!" This was the reply of a naive nursing student. I hadn't seen many wounds yet. I had no idea what the parameters of the medical arts were. He said they were going to save his leg, and I was thrilled for him. I later learned they hadn't told him yet. Stephen was dead set on saving his leg. The doctors felt it was already lost.

Stephen smiled reassuringly to me, "It's a tough leg to work on. Most of the nurses pull up a chair and sit down, because it takes a while to do." I followed his suggestion. I pulled up a chair, and with Stephen's help, we changed his dressing. Together we re-read the directions, talking and problem-solving our way through it. I scrupulously maintained my sterile technique. Stephen cheered me on along the way. "Yeah, that's good, just like that, nice."

Forty-five minutes later we were through. Stephen complemented me on a job well done. But I am sure I was much more impressed with him than he was with me. I thought about how I would feel looking down at my own beloved leg and seeing it in shreds. I thought about how I felt when I first saw my appendectomy scar, the pain that I felt when I realized my belly would never look the same. The scar is only slightly visible now, but I still resent it's presence.

A three inch scar is a very small price to pay for being alive, but it is a price. I multiplied how I felt times the enormity of damage to Stephen's leg. The sorrow at seeing your own flesh mangled is a very personal thing. Stephen didn't talk about that part of it, and I didn't ask. The sadness that I felt for my patients was hard to tolerate, so I turned it into anger. Motorcycles were a wonderful target. The most maiming injuries on the unit were always motorcycles. The machine turned healthy limbs into bare bones and shredded muscles. Motorcycles created mutilated limbs that I couldn't look upon without feeling tremendous anguish for the owner. I left infected ortho with an unbridled hatred for motorcycles.

I fell into the routine with everyone else on the unit. There were some jobs I liked, some I hated. Handing out medications and hanging IV's were the two jobs on the unit that could only be performed by an RN or a senior nursing student. Because almost every patient was on intravenous antibiotics Cheryl had received special permission in using her own protocol in hanging IV's. Most units hang only one bottle at a time. But on infected ortho the entire day's worth of medications were hung at once. One nurse was assigned to monitoring all IV's during a shift. The IV nurse began first thing in the morning collecting orders and preparing and labeling all the solutions before making rounds of the patients.

We were each assigned to the job of IV's for a week. The first day we observed, the second day we helped, the third day we were observed. Once the solutions were prepared we loaded up a large cart and made the rounds of the unit. At each bedside the lines were checked for patency, and problem IV's were restarted. Normal saline was kept dripping all day, and at the prescribed times antibiotics were run in also. This job made me nervous because there was such a small margin for error. A mistake could be quickly disastrous.

Before being allowed to take pediatrics, all student nurses had to pass a medication math test. This was to be sure we could figure out children's doses based on their weight, make conversions where needed, and establish the rate of flow of an IV. We were given a formula to determine amount of fluid per minute and hour that was entering a patient's veins. We were told that this formula was one of those little mysteries of nursing, still as yet undiscovered by M.D.'s. It would be our responsibility to make sure all of the IV's were flowing at the prescribed rate, especially if we had seen some doctor fiddling with them. We were also encouraged to try to teach willing doctors the formula. But, they warned us, willing doctors would be rare, and teaching them would not be easy.

This proved to be true. I found only one willing doctor, and he became tired of the process by step three, saying, "it's easier to guestimate it." I joined the ranks of concerned nurses carefully adjusting IV's after doctors had messed with them.

I worried about many things when I was the IV nurse. I worried that I would forget a cross-check, or that somehow I would hang the wrong bottle and run it into a patient's veins. This is not an unrealistic worry because these things happen and patients do die. I checked everything, rechecked, and checked again. I would try to focus my mind for eight hours on every detail of the IV's. These were not steps that I had performed enough that they were automatically imbedded in my brain. I had to constantly concentrate to make sure there were no screw-ups while I administered and monitored IV antibiotics to thirty-five patients. This was why there were no relief nurses floated to this unit. Cheryl wanted to work only with staff she had trained and who were familiar with the procedures.

By the end of the week I was proclaimed competent by the supervising IV nurse. From then on, I was assigned IV's all by myself on a regular basis. It was the same for all four of the students working this unit. I would spend the shift maintaining my focus, doing everything I could to prevent foul-ups. Afterwards, I would return to my dorm room, strip, grab some devil's food cookies, and veg out to Mary Tyler Moore reruns. She became my after work retreat. I would lie on the bed with my feet up, moving only enough to convey chocolate cookies and milk to my mouth. One hour of back to back old MTM shows, and I had recovered enough to shower and join the world.

Passing out medications was the other job that could only be performed by an RN or a senior student. The nurse assigned meds for the day was handed the keys to the medication room. Medications on every unit are kept locked up. Infected orthopedics, like surgical units, involved so much pain that a good percent of the meds given were narcotics. Because of the potential for abuse by both staff and patients, narcotics require more involved documentation than other medications.

The medical perspective on the administration of narcotics is constantly evolving. During the sixties the potential for abuse became much more apparent, and doctors became hesitant to over-medicate their patients. The use of pain medication is an emotion-laden subject. Doctors, nurses - everyone - has an opinion, and it is frequently laced as much with emotion as it is with rational thinking. As students nurses we studied the literature on the use of narcotics for pain control. Researchers were finding a significant drop in cases of post-surgical pneumonia when patients were medicated for pain and then encouraged to get out of bed and start walking around.

Other articles noted that pain was much easier to control and responded to smaller doses of medication, if one medicated earlier, and more frequently (every three hours instead of every four). The theory was to control the pain at its onset with codeine rather than waiting until it became intense and required a stronger narcotic like Demerol. I believe with more recent research, and with the current anti-drug focus, that the medical community has taken another swing back to a more conservative approach with narcotics. There has also been the introduction of new non-narcotic drugs available for short-term pain control. For chronic pain, people are turning more recently to biofeedback and mental imaging as an alternative to medication.

As a nurse who hated dealing with pain, I had a special affinity for the job of medication nurse. Most medications are ordered by the medical doctor in a format that includes dosage and frequency. Orders for pain medication are written up a little differently. Here the drug and the amount are specified, but the frequency is usually listed as every three to four hours, PRN. PRN means the medication is given only if the patient requests it. The theory is you don't want to be medicating patients unless they are in enough pain to request it. I had some problems with this protocol when I put it into practice.

The majority of meds were given out three times a day. At eight o'clock, noon, and four o'clock the medication nurse made rounds of the unit passing out what was ordered. This is not a quick procedure. It usually takes twenty to thirty minutes to prepare and pour meds for thirty-five patients. Patients may be receiving up to a dozen medications beyond what is hanging in their IV's. Medical science can create some amazing cocktails. Once the meds are prepared, the cart is also loaded up with orange juice, ready for bedside delivery.

An efficient nurse is going to take about half an hour to dispense the meds. A nurse playing the hostess with the mostest such as myself, needed a full hour. I liked this job; it was so clean and pleasant. I would roll my shiny stainless steel cart along, beaming warm sociability. I can't help it. My mother and father are marvelous hosts. I had spent a lifetime observing my gracious parents welcoming people into their home with casual elegance. I am marked with it as if it were an indelible ink. Place a silver tray in front of me, and I am compelled to smile and serve with charm and grace.

Our patients from the barrio and ghettos must have found me pretty entertaining. Most nurses would move quickly through them, passing out their meds with some friendly chatter or a snide retort. I resembled something along the lines of Princess Di making a visit. Head high, face shinning, tall and slim, I would enter the room to share my treats with everyone. I must have appeared as an escapee from Wonderland as I slowly worked my way through the room, visiting with each one, handing out my little gift of drugs.

My morning medication rounds would not be completed until almost nine o'clock. By ten o'clock the patients' dressing changes were underway or completed. This meant if I wanted to get patients medicated for pain before their dressing changes, I really had to hustle. Almost half of the pain meds given on our unit were given as injections. We did not have the unit dosage syringes that are available today. All injected medication had to be drawn up in the syringe, sometimes requiring reconstituting from powder. Narcotics require extra paperwork, and all this took time. Medication injected into the muscle requires about twenty minutes to take effect. Therefore, timing was important. If I waited for each patient to individually request their pain meds, many would be in severe pain for almost an hour after their dressings were changed.

By my second day as medication nurse I had begun a new system for myself. Along with my pleasant bedside visit and drug delivery to each patient, I would also ask those with serious wounds if they would be needing some pain medication before their dressing change. This is a questionable act. One is not supposed to offer PRN meds to patients, unless they request it first. Patients are very smart. They caught the unusual routine immediately. The nurse from Wonderland strikes again. "Why yes, thank you, I would like something for my pain." Frequently, they would then make requests, often for medications stronger than the ones ordered for them. I gave each patient the meds prescribed for them, but realized my system was flawed and would require modification.

I was not consistent in my attitude regarding regulations. Though I had been flexible in my approach to delivering pain meds, Mr. Charley Jones was a patient who discovered an area where I was very rigid. Charley was here because he had an accident years ago that had left him with a chronic bone infection, osteomyelitis, that would never really clear up. Intermittently he would have to be re-admitted to Infected Ortho. to receive IV antibiotics. The antibiotics would temporarily make the infection back off. What he really needed was surgery, but his hypertension was so bad, none of the doctors felt his body would survive the added stress of an operation.

Mr. Jones was in his mid-forties, large-boned, broad-shouldered, and obese. Charley liked women, drink, and food. His attitude towards life was one of lustful appreciation. His huge chest provided a laugh or an angry roar that would resonate throughout the unit. Like many otherwise healthy black men, diet, stress, and genetics had combined to create severe hypertension. Charley's blood pressure would have looked fine as a batting average, but it was a poor prognosis for longevity.

Charley was a charismatic man who appeared bent on doing himself in. He had an interesting array of women visitors. Young, pretty, black women, wearing tight short skirts, high heels, and low cut-tops usually came in two's and sometimes in three's. They would take him for rides in a wheelchair, or hang over the sides of his bed, leaning on his large belly. Sometimes they would get up in the bed with him, two or three of them laughing and teasing.

These were really girls, not women, most of them were under twenty-one, and they obviously adored Charley. All the girls were like darling pets for him; he didn't appear to like one any better than the others. They took turns kissing and petting with Charley, doing their nails and talking nonsense in their off moments. There was a sense of family in this group. I would join this voluptuous crowd and visit with everyone in my little white cap and my stiff uniform collapsing on my chest. The girls would sneak in every form of candy and salty snack for Charley, everything that was sure to kill him. I would describe in detail the physiological implication of these snacks on Mr. Jones' body; I even would draw pictures for them. I thought the girls were just lacking the knowledge to understand the implications of their actions. I would hover around the perimeter of this circle of tight skirts, patterned stockings, and bouffant hair trying to share with them my understanding of hypertension and its effects on the kidneys of the man they loved.

In retrospect, I see his family a little differently. I see what was probably a pimp with his girls, who were devoted and would do anything for a man who could be teasing and sweet, or angry and mean. If Charley had wanted pure buckets of salt from the sea, these girls would have brought them to him. My lectures and diagrams were nonsense in the face of meeting Mr. Jones' immediate needs. These girls would probably risk their own lives before disappointing Charley.

I enjoyed talking with Charley between visiting hours whenever I was assigned to his room. Between bed baths and dressing changes, I would draw pictures of his entrails, trying once again to explain his disease to him. We would also talk and argue politics, economics and life in general.

Very near the end of my rotation on Infected Ortho I was cleaning up around Mr. Jones. I had opened up the drawer next to his bed to put away his thermometer, and I found an entire storehouse of pharmaceuticals. He had a rainbow collection of pills in bottles, and none of it was stuff we were passing out to him on the unit. I realized that Charley's girls were bringing him more than salt and sugar. To me this was serious. His recreational drug use was his own business, but I figured Charley could accidentally kill himself mixing this stuff with the potent cocktail the doctors were already giving him.

I explained this to Charley. I told him the medications he was on were dangerous enough, and that mixing them with his own stuff was really risky. Mr. Jones grew dark and growled at me, "Fuck you, stay out of my business, this has nothing to do with you." The intensity and heat coming from him was intimidating. He tensed like a man who could kill. My survival instincts immediately backed me off. No more words were exchanged, and I left his room.

There was a choice to be made. Charley had made his. He would take what ever drugs he pleased. Now I could be silent and honor his decision, or I could attempt to intervene. If I hadn't heard his big loud laugh and seen the warmth in him, I might have been able to act differently, but I can't say for sure. He had frightened me, but I still cared about him. I went to Cheryl and told her. Cheryl's face turned tired and sagged as she saw the intensity in mine. She tried to avoid what I was requiring of her. She said some patients will just do as they please; and this is true. But I couldn't accept it. "He could die Cheryl, and we could have prevented it."

What ever her personal feelings may have been, I had left Cheryl no ethical choice. In the face of a naive student nurse, struggling for a patient's life, she had to go by the rules, even if they did not fit the reality of Charley Jones. She told me not to worry about it, or to bother Mr. Jones, she would take care of it. Cheryl is an ethical woman; shoulders tired and slumped she went in to deal with Mr. Jones. His drugs were confiscated and Charley Jones was mad as hell.

Strategically Cheryl never assigned me to Charley again. I would see him though, when passing out medications or IV's. He didn't let it slide. He told me I was a pain in the butt, a rat, a fink, and a snitch. I repeated for him my reasons for turning him in. Charley tolerated me after that, but the warmth was absolutely gone. He never forgave me. When I was about to graduate, I told Charley I had to go take a final exam. He said he hoped I failed, and I knew he meant it. The pain of his last remark lingers still.

Violating another's personal rights in order to "protect" them is an extremely difficult decision. I almost always stand on the side of personal rights. I feel I truly did violate Charley Jones. If presented with the dilemma today my actions would probably be different. The more I come to know myself and others the greater my respect for the rights of each of us to make our own life decisions.

We were one third of the way through our last semester of nursing school. It was now time to change units. Next Monday I would show up on Neuro Med and once again assume the position of the neophyte. Just about the time we became confident and self-assured on a unit it was time to move on. Cheryl told us we were welcome back for team leading or after graduation as a part of the staff. I knew I wouldn't be back after graduation and I hadn't made up my mind yet about team leading. I was waiting to see what kind of surprises Neuro Med held for me.

I admired and respected Cheryl South. I thought she probably worked too hard and may have traded a personal life for a professional one, but she was a wonderful nurse. I left the goo and the gore, hoping never to return to it. All the time I was aware that even the goo of infected orthopedics might be better than Neuro Med, so I might chose the lesser of two evils and come back for our final rotation, team leading. We toasted good bye to the "pus ward" with popcorn and Coke in the nurses' lounge and turned our thoughts to the coma patients on Neuro Med.

Chapter Twenty-Four

Mindless Movement

Towards the latter part of nursing school Jeff and I were spending every weekend together. Our relationship had developed to the point that he had given me a bottom drawer in his closet to leave a few of my things in. This is a specific step in a relationship. This can be a pragmatic move made with much intellectual discussion, or it can be made in a swell of romantic affection. This step is a milestone; it makes a statement. The message is, "I am going to allow you to leave some things in my home. Things that will remind me of you in your absence and will take up some of my precious space. These are things that I will have to explain, should someone else look in that drawer." It also says, "This space in my home belongs to you." It is a space that will have to be relinquished by one and reclaimed by the other, should the relationship terminate. It is a complication in one's life, to give up a drawer to another.

Jeff and I undertook this step in a rather unconscious manner. One day, he opened a drawer, and pulled out his clothes. "Why don't you keep some of your things in here, so you don't have to lug everything back and forth all the time." My stomach tensed a little. I thought about it. He was making such a generous offer. I was aware of the implications of taking up drawer space in Jeff's home. I didn't think about it too much, though. I didn't want to stress our relationship with excessive insight. "How romantic," I thought, "a drawer in the closet. Absolutely, all right, I'll put some things in here." And so we began our tentative steps forward into the land of monogamy and commitment.

During my last semester at County, the weather was turning warm. Sunshine for Jeff meant the beach. Jeff thrives on the Southern California beaches and their ambiance. Body surfing, skateboarding, and rollerskating were his sports. The forest and horses were my loves, but I had put those activities on hold for a while because the only animals in the trees at County were rats, and horses were too expensive.

Jeff preferred Venice Beach. The atmosphere there was like a circus, with constant partying and exhibitionism. The colorful craziness invigorated and enlivened him. The artist in his soul connected with the freedom of expression that abounds in Venice. I am a voyeur and sociologist by nature. I loved observing the action at Venice Beach.

So I was not an unhappy companion, climbing out of bed early every Saturday morning and heading to the beach before the air had begun to warm. We were off for sun and roller-skating. I didn't tell Jeff how I really felt about roller-skating. Roller-skating is enjoyable in moderation, just for fun. Moderation was not a term in Jeff's vocabulary. He was more an all-out kind of person. People like that think moderation is sort of wimpy.

Jeff loved to skate. When he and I were becoming friends, he would talk about Bonnie, his girlfriend at that time. He felt she didn't really share his love of skating. She had taken a bad fall, landing hard on her bottom. That seemed to have slowed down her enthusiasm for the sport. I could believe it; a fall on the tailbone is not good. At the time Bonnie's birthday was approaching and Jeff was debating her present. He really wanted to buy her skates, but he had a feeling she would prefer a necklace. He had asked my opinion, what should he get her. I told him if he wanted to please her, get her the necklace.

Bonnie got the necklace, and their relationship flourished. Two and a half years later it was my turn. For my twenty-eighth birthday, I got the skates. I saw the irony in this, but I let it go. Actually, I didn't get the skates, I got the wheels. Jeff was a thrifty sort of man. He said he knew I would just love some skates, so for my birthday, he would buy me the wheels and I could pay for the boots and fittings to hold the wheels. Granted, these were expensive wheels. Super fast, state of the art, go like the wind, fall down and kill yourself wheels.

I had learned to skate at five years old. In a whoosh I could swoop under the Ping-Pong table. I could go fast. I could turn. I couldn't skate backwards or jump curbs, and stopping was tricky. I did all this on normal old steel wheels. Jeff gave me the wonder wheels of the moment. If you inhaled you went forward, in you exhaled you went backwards. My wheels were faster than the speed of thought. I was totally out of control. Jeff was so hyped with my new skates he was ready to fly. We were off to the boardwalk at Venice Beach, to skate with the primo skaters of them all. We were going to dance on our skates with all the cool black guys. We would rip along the boardwalk in our bathing suits, jumping the curbs, the salt air in our noses. We would become the local color.

Jeff was crazy, but not a reckless crazy. Besides the wheels, he had also given me wrists guards. If I fell it was OK, my wrists would not be fractured. I could slide safely along the pavement on my plastic wrist guards. This was not consoling to a woman exposing great expanses of skin in a tiny string bikini. We pulled Jeff's truck into the beach parking lot and sat on the bumper. Here we casually tied uncontrollable contraptions of speed onto our feet. Up to this point, I had been in denial. "This is OK, we can go slow. I can handle this." I had tried the skates out previously on the kitchen linoleum, and had nearly crashed and burned. Jeff assured me they would be slower on pavement.

The moment I stood, my denial dissipated, and I knew I was in trouble. These skates scared the shit out of me, and Jeff was already off, cruising twenty yards ahead of me. I wobbled on my legs like a newborn colt, taking tiny choppy steps. Jeff finally noticed I had not whooshed to his side, and came back to retrieve me. It was time to realign our fantasies closer to reality. Jeff altered his expectations from immediate skating champion to she'll catch on quickly and in a couple of weeks she'll be able to start doing some dance steps.

I went in the other direction. I thought to myself, he'll understand this is tough and he will take pleasure in skating slowly with me. I had rosy pictures of us rolling along the boardwalk at a gentle speed, soaking in the scenery, enjoying the sunshine. I explained I was more of a cruising skater than a dancing skater. Jeff made an effort to meet me halfway. The first hour or two we would skate along the boardwalk. But we went in the direction of the crowds, and we did it quickly. What probably felt like crawling to him was flying to me. We sped through throngs of babies, dogs, bicycles, cars and wildly clad people. We rushed through narrow lanes lined with vendors' booths and shoppers. We skirted spilled ice cream cones and dog poop. Just when I would begin to feel like I might survive, we would come to a curb.

Jeff flew off the curbs with a beautiful long jump, his face one beaming, confident smile. I began to die a little as I saw the curb approaching. Cars would rush past, with people crowding and pushing, and the curb would loom closer and closer. I would try to break my speed. I would attempt a snow plow. I never dared use the rubber stopper on the front of the skates, which seemed like a death tool if ever I had seen one. I was sure if I hit that stopper while I was still moving I would flatten my face on the pavement. I would slow myself to the speed of an infant's crawl. A yard from the curb I would turn my body parallel to it. Then I would cautiously approach the edge, side stepping. My long arms would wave madly, to help me maintain my balance. My bikini bottoms would hike up the cheeks of my fanny. I had the first unplanned thong bathing suit. I would cautiously step off the curb.

One foot down, one foot up, I would wobble like crazy. If I adjusted my suit now, I would land in the gutter. An ungraceful clomp brought the other skate down to rest in the street. By this time Jeff's head would have disappeared into the crowd. Alone, I would flail my way across a street riddled with pot holes and traffic. The ascension on the other side was easier. I had built up no speed. I just had to clomp my way up the other curb. Finally, I could pull my bathing suit bottoms back down, and precede with some modicum of dignity. Jeff would be pulled up somewhere waiting for me. He would be listening to a musician or watching a mime. Wearing only his bathing suit, Jeff was a tall, tan, beautiful beacon of health. After an hour of skating behind him, my ego had sunk so low you would have needed sonar to find it.

Having put in his "quality time" with me, Jeff was now free to really enjoy himself. Our towels were carefully laid out on the sand right next to the parking lot. This is where Hank, and his dancing friends, always parked their van. The back doors were swung open, and Hank would drag out two three foot speakers. Disco and soul screamed from the machine. The alcohol was poured into plastic cups to make it look like soft drinks. Once they had enough booze on board, the men began. They skated slowly at first, taking long glides, stretching out to the music. First the feet, then the thighs and hips, would catch the rhythm. Finally the arms, the neck, and the head would fall into the flow. Soft, easy moves, loose and fluid, the world and the mind displaced by music and motion.

Jeff wouldn't join them yet, the time wasn't right. We would sit by the side and watch, as the dancers moved from cool to warm. There was a pause once they were warm, a little more booze, and the clothes began to come off. Bare chest, bare legs, only sun glasses and shorts were left, as a perfect black torso began to spin. Only the guys with the really stunning bodies stripped down. Hank was about forty and paunchy. However, when he chose, he was a tremendous dancer. He wore a T-shirt and jeans, and a navy watch cap on his head. His spins were incredibly tight, his legs were lightning, but his endurance was shot. The joy of the dance had dimmed for him; now it was alcohol and girls. He provided the alcohol and the music, the young beautiful men provided the girls.

This is where Jeff fit in. He was allowed to hang out and dance because he was competent, and he looked good. His skating was not on a par with these guys, but he was well-built and white. A day in the sun was long and Hank liked variety. He loved the beautiful black girls in hot pink and lime green micro-bikinis. He also liked a few white chicks sprinkled in too, preferably thirsty blondes with big breasts. Jeff was just right for Hank's needs. He didn't drink, so he was an easy keeper. He couldn't outdance the black guys, so he wasn't any competition, and white girls felt more comfortable hanging around with one white guy present.

Jeff had been dancing with Hank and his friends every weekend for a year or so when I first began skating with him. I was not considered a great addition. I was tolerated as a courtesy to Jeff. I was of no use in attracting admiring females. I didn't drink with Hank, so I was of no entertainment value, and as all but Jeff could see, my dancing on skates was hopeless. I would sit around acting the loving groupie, for about thirty minutes. Finally, the cool treatment from the gang and the repetitious music would wear down my patience. I would then move on to the skating I enjoyed.

Each Saturday, while Jeff danced with Hank and the guys, I would put on my shorts and take off down the bike path. I wouldn't travel in our earlier direction, but head north. A clear open path stretched for miles, with no curbs, no streets, and no crowds. I would take long, smooth strides, rolling along at a leisurely pace. I thought skating would be the perfect way to see the world. As long as there were no curbs, no streets, no hills, and all was perfect smoothness. Traveling at my own pace, I felt confident and alive. I even felt beautiful as I watched my leg muscles defining and redefining themselves in the sun. My head came up, I no longer studied the pavement for cracks. I became bigger, stronger, more powerful as I skated, enjoying my body and the hot sun.

Jeff and I had a ritual. After a day at the beach, we would spend the late afternoon house hunting. It was a strange ritual for two people who had not officially decided to get married. I guess people who decide to live together long term do this, but that wasn't exactly us either. I am not sure what was exactly us, because we didn't directly discuss it. Instead, we talked about what type of house we wanted to buy. The unstated meaning being, we would live there together. The unstated meaning was also, we would get married.

Since we weren't engaged, and we didn't talk about when we might choose to get engaged or married, things were a little confusing to say the least. Who was buying this house? Were we buying it as a couple, or was Jeff buying it alone? Was this our dream home, where we would raise our family? Was Jeff planning to bring a roommate? Would there be several roommates, like he had at the present? I don't know what I was thinking. For an incredibly opinionated person, I acted like I was devoid of thought.

We would look at a home and I would think, "This is not bad, I could live here." Jeff would look at the same house, and say, "I like this, but the price is too high. It's a good thing I could rent out the two back bedrooms." One bathroom, three men, and me, sounds like personal hygiene hell to me. Jeff's roommates were always art students. Young, interesting, creative, sloppy, unbearably messy men. Young men prepping for a date take at least two hours in the bathroom. They are not above panicking at the last minute and redoing the whole thing. Young males are darling to watch, fun to listen to, and a real pain to live with. They are not much different from young women. I found this out living with Jeff's roommates on the weekends. Acne meds, shaving cream, hair gel, hair spray, blemish cover-up sticks, deodorant, and cologne covered every available space in the bathroom. This is all fine as a novelty, but as a way of life, I preferred a bathroom free of young men.

While Jeff counted the number of possible roommates he could squeeze in, I was thinking, "this house is a little too large." This was a silent play on my part. As the darling little mute, I would not give voice to my feelings. With every moment of silence, I was creating impassable chasms for us to deal with later.

One reason for my silence was that I had accepted the myth of timetables. There are times during which one is most likely to find a mate. I somehow felt that if I got past a crucial mating period without finding a partner, I would be alone. Being permanently single was never one of my fantasies. I hadn't gone to nursing school to get married. I had gone there to become a nurse. In the recesses of my heart and mind, there was a hidden agenda I hadn't shared with anyone, even myself. It was the secret of wanting a love, a romance, a lifetime mate. My exposure to males while in nursing school was high. By the time I had acknowledged to myself my desire to find a mate, my time in school was quickly coming to a close.

I think Jeff and I had both reached a time in our lives where we were ready for a sense of permanence and belonging, and there we were, right in each other's arms. Time spent together was fun, warm, and playful. I loved the creative aspect of his career. I have always been independent and have needed private time to myself. It seemed perfect to me that Jeff spent so much time working. I would have plenty of time alone. Together we painted a picture of our future that looked good to both of us.

In retrospect, it seems Jeff and I had a clearer idea of our future than we did of our present. It saddens me that I didn't know what was going on inside Jeff's head through all of this. I didn't know his fears or private concerns. I think we often do know the major traps lying ahead for each of us. I believe we usually choose not to think about them. At least this is true for me. If I had been very honest with myself, I would have admitted that Jeff and I were having some serious discrepancies in our house hunting.

The hunt for our house went on for months. It became one of our pastimes. We combed the streets of our favorite towns once a week, for about seven months. We didn't find our perfect home until three months after I graduated from nursing school. When we found it, it was true love for both of us. A big old house, really old, on a big old lot, really big, and every part of it was completely run down and in disrepair. We were in a wonderful, quiet town. From our bedroom windows we could see the snowy cap of Mt. Baldy, and the run-off from the mountains trickled through the tail end of our backyard.

Getting to that point was an adventure, much of it painful. I remember many details of that time, but one day is vivid beyond the others. That one day should have told me a number of truths, but I was not yet ready to listen. For school or life to be a teacher, the learner must be ready for the lesson and paying close attention. It is clear to me that I was not ready to learn these lessons then. It is a gift I give to myself, to learn them now, rather than to lose them completely.

On a warm day in late May, Jeff and I had skated through our morning at the beach, and I had a slight burn. We were in his hand-built hot rod truck, The Amana, named (by me) because it looked like a white refrigerator. We were headed toward the northern part of town, where property was much less expensive. It was one of those areas that had become completely run down. The windows wore bars. People parked their cars on the lawn, and put their old car seats on the front porch to sit in and drink beer, partying their way through the hot summer nights.

It was also a segregated neighborhood. First, it had belonged to the whites, and then it had proceeded through the cycle that neighborhoods go through all around big cities. I never saw it when it was a lovely neighborhood, but all the signs were there to indicate it had once been. I didn't see any of its phases and cycles. I only saw it's present state, ten years ago. By that time, white people were no longer welcome. Other colors of people were tolerated more. I assume there was a descending rainbow of colors of desirability, with white taking up last place. Therefore, true to form, liberal whites had decided this was the perfect next location for gentrification. I love that word; the pomposity of it dazzles me. The up and coming young whites were going to buy the only houses they could afford, fix them up and hopefully drive the current residents as far away from the neighborhood as possible.

The very fringes of this neighborhood were just beginning to be encroached upon by young yuppies with babies in arms. These were the areas Jeff and I occasionally prowled. He felt this was where we would eventually be. I was worried. Security bars were everywhere, and rottweilers stood guard behind five foot fences surrounding entire properties. We talked to some residents in the neighborhood, "How do you like living here?" We were told property prices were good. "My wife loves the house. She won't go out in the front yard alone, but she loves the house. The dogs make it a lot safer." I was not charmed. The idea of living where I was not wanted, sounded very unappealing.

Jeff and I had spent twenty minutes or so cruising this neighborhood that we were beginning to know fairly well. He thought the prices were still too high here, and that we needed to get a little more adventurous. So we drove farther north about ten blocks. We were now in an area that never had any pretense of old charm. The streets were tightly lined with small two bedroom houses on dirt lots. Residents had gone from security bars to full encampment. The air was tense. Hostile glances followed our truck as we slowly wound our way through the grim, hot streets. Jeff noted here it was a good thing we brought the truck. "Your convertible bug looks so yuppie, we might not be welcome."

I didn't think carrying a white flag was going to do us any good at this point. But I was being tolerant. I was going to keep my mouth shut as we cruised this DMZ. I knew Jeff was thrifty, but I figured he couldn't be this far over the edge. It wasn't bad, though I was a little frightened we would be victims of a drive by shooting. But I was hanging in there. And then we saw the sign, FOR SALE BY OWNER. Jeff lit up all teeth and shining eyes. I slumped farther into the seat, "You don't want to stop, do you?"

Of course he wanted to stop. This was great. Jeff was sure he could afford this house. It was the tiniest house on the street, about two hundred square feet. The lot was long and narrow, with a few patches of crab grass clinging tenaciously to the arid dirt of the front yard. We parked the truck and Jeff hopped out, tall, tan, and blond, dressed in white shorts, grinning like a victorious tennis player. I followed behind in my brief beach shorts, tank top, and matching sun hat. My outfit looked darling on the beach, and suicidal in the ghetto.

We trotted up to the front door in our perfect running shoes. Jeff was eager to explore his next possible home. Heavy steel grills were bolted onto the windows from the inside. The cost of bars must have been prohibitive. If this house caught on fire you would fry inside. The sign had said open and the door was ajar, so Jeff walked right in; reluctantly, I followed. There was a man on his hands and knees working on the flooring. He stood to greet us. He was a tall attractive, well groomed man, like a black version of Jeff. This pleased Jeff to no end. He turned to me and gave a smug smile, as if to say, "See, I told you this was a perfectly good neighborhood."

"Hello," Jeff was beaming, "we're interested in buying this house. Do you live here?" The man looked at us, as if he had been spit upon. "I would never live here, I just own it. My wife and I live in South Pasadena." "Lucky woman," I thought.

"Well we're thinking of living here. How's the neighborhood, it looks pretty nice?" By now, the man was looking at Jeff in total disbelief. He then looked at me, searching my face for signs of craziness too. What he saw was a woman who couldn't believe she was with such an asshole. Apparently he had seen this expression on a woman's face before. He shook his head and rolled his eyes. He let me know this was my problem, that he wouldn't save me. He proceeded to ignore Jeff and I completely. Jeff chattered on about the wonders of the house, but to this man's mind, we no longer existed.

We proceed to "tour" the house, which required us to rotate in a one hundred and eighty degree circle. We had now seen the house. This was not enough. Jeff was serious about this. He had sold his antique MG a week ago for several thousand dollars; that, combined with his savings, gave him twelve thousand dollars. He was excited because he could actually buy this house straight out cash, all by himself. So we took a more in-depth look at the house. This required us to take six paces in each direction to see the three other rooms. The bedroom was a transformed closet and was exactly the size of a twin bed mattress.

After seeing the bedroom my mind began to fog over. I have blocked out the kitchen and bathroom completely from my memory. This was probably a little kindness my mind performed for me. Jeff poked his head out the back door and then pulled it back in. He told the man, "We want to walk around and absorb the neighborhood."

I was slipping into one of those surreal moments where the person I was with and knew so well seemed like a complete stranger. Certainly, nothing could have been stranger than Jeff's behavior at that moment. I have more sympathy for him now. A bargain shopper like myself knows the allure of something so major being affordable. That may have been why panic gripped my stomach. I knew the seduction of being able to afford what was presumed unaffordable. In this case, it was a house, a horrid little terrible house, but a house. I remembered the piles of things I have purchased in my life, inappropriate, unnecessary things, whose prices were too tantalizing to resist. "God, I'm doomed. Jeff is going to buy this house."

In a numbed state, I followed Jeff out of doors to, "absorb the neighborhood." Jeff closed his eyes and stretched out his limbs. He truly made an effort to absorb the vibrations of this place. I was not so adventurous. To me the vibrations felt toxic. I withdrew inside myself, sealing up my pores so the hostility in the air couldn't seep in. A wadded up little me followed a few paces behind the wide open flowering Jeff as we began to explore.

There is not much to see in a narrow dirt back yard. We proceeded to the back gate and opened it. "Attractive alley", narrow, dirty, trash cans overflowing, your basic alley. Jeff saw my face and responded, "We could put a lock on this gate." "Good idea." We reversed our direction, traversing the little yard, to walk along the side of the house, past two windows and more steel mesh, to the front yard. Jeff spread his arms, lifted his hands palms up and began to breathe deeply. I knew what he was doing. He was inhaling the neighborhood, absorbing it into his lungs. My mind is flexible so Jeff's behavior did not weird me out.

A high pitched shout issued from the house next door. A woman's voice screaming obscenities like a flame thrower set the air on fire. A deep man's voice bellowed in return. But she was the stronger. I could feel her strength in the heat of her anger. The intensity of her anger expelled him from the house. His pride was hurt. His temper was building, but his couldn't match hers. She followed him out, and the fight continued. The hate and pain were overflowing. There were no words mean enough to vent their feelings. The pitch intensified.

She screeched, he boomed. His big booming did not quell her a bit. She stood firm, seething. I believed she would kill him, if he did not retreat. He must have seen it my way. Huge, boiling with anger, he retreated.

His car was parked at the curb. Still shouting and swearing, he drove off. Finally, I took a breath. I looked over at Jeff. His open flower had transformed into a hard protective shell. We got into his truck quickly. If there was to be a round two, we did not want to be present. We drove several blocks before I realized I was soaked in sweat. It was tense and shocking, but I couldn't resist, I had to say it, "Nice neighborhood, I guess they'd be our neighbors." I thought I had gotten through it with a glib retort, but then began to shake and cry uncontrollably." I don't want to live there. I love you, but why do I have to be miserable because I love you? I am not a snob, I just don't want to live there."

Jeff was angry with me. I don't remember his argument. It was based on the usual things that came up between us. This was a house he could afford all by himself, cash. I was being unsupportive, and acting spoiled. I sat there quietly not defending or explaining my feelings. I look back now, and I see me shaken by one woman's explosion of anger. A total unleashing of feelings seems purging next to my pent up little squeak of anger. This woman was terrifying and hypnotizing to me. She had let loose her feelings and the earth had not opened up and swallowed her. The man had left and whether she liked it or not, he would probably be back.

It was a while before Jeff and I hit the house hunting trail again. Once we did our searching moved farther and farther south until we landed in a neighborhood we could both feel comfortable with. We did not speak about the little house again. Jeff and I never did sit down and talk about what each of us wanted in our relationship or in our home. We continued to go forward with mindless movement; ignoring the small cracks that spread out around us like fault lines with every step we took.

Chapter Twenty-Five

Tending The Garden

I entered the Neurological Medicine unit holding onto the positive thought, "I am almost through nursing school!" I clung to this soothing thought because the forward press on Neuro Med was not good. I had heard an upper level student refer to it as the garden, because all of his patients were vegetables. Nearly all of the patients on this unit were in a coma, or in some level of semi-conscious state. My friend spoke in terms of feeding, suctioning, and turning his patients regularly on the hour. All of the vegetables were in neat little rows in his garden.

As a highly verbal psycho-social nurse, I was not looking forward to a series of coma cases. Everyone would be fully tubed, with nasogastric tubes for eating, catheters for urinating, occasionally IV's, and frequently tracheotomies with respirators attached. Suctioning out respirators was my least favorite thing to do in the whole world. Respiratory mucus is one of those things that can just get you down.

Gilbert assigned me my first patient, a young Chinese man named Tam. He had been in an auto accident several weeks ago, and was now semicomatose, which meant with effort he could be aroused. Tam lay small, delicate, and very still in his bed. He had a tracheotomy with a respirator in his throat. His eyes were taped shut, so they wouldn't stay open and dry out, since he had lost his reflex to blink. The catheter bag attached to his bed was half full.

The thing I first noticed most about Tam was the way he held his body. He lay straight, but very pulled in, tight, and tense looking. The room felt chilly to me, so I asked him if he was cold. People on respirators can not speak, so I don't know what type of response I was expecting. I put my hands on Tam's face, and I introduced myself. I touched his arms, legs, and feet, and decided he felt cold. I hunted down a couple of extra blankets to covered him up, and that is how I began working with patients in comas.

Tam was not completely unconscious. He could intermittently respond to yes or no questions by squeezing my hand. It took me a little while to discover this. I would have to watch very carefully as I worked with him, for the different small signs of his responsiveness. As I washed Tam's face that morning I could see a small sliver of his eyes through the strips of tape. I stuck my head down like a curious chicken and peeked inside. My face was an inch from his, "Tam, can you see me, can you see me out here?" No response.

Nothing on Tam's chart indicated that he was aware of what was going on around him. So I had to discover him, piece by piece, by myself. I was a determined ferret as I set about trying to see if Tam could interact with me. I wasn't trying to save Tam, I was trying to save me. I needed patients with whom I could communicate. Feedback was my goal. I was sure I could see a glint in his eyes. If he was in there, I wanted him to talk to me.

Tam had very little control of his body. For the most part he was a limp doll. I discovered his small amount of hand control by putting my finger in his hand and telling him to squeeze. "Squeeze my finger Tam, squeeze my finger." I immediately felt disappointment that Tam's hand remained inert. I started thinking what else I could try. Yelling louder crossed my mind, in case I hadn't gotten his attention. My mind was so busy racing around, searching for other possibilities, it took me a moment to notice a small tickling sensation on my hand. Tam was attempting to squeeze it.

Tam taught me several things about patients in comas. I learned that semicomatose patients do not respond quickly. If I wanted to communicate with Tam, I would have to be patient, and look for slow, incremental responses. At the touch of Tam's fingers, I swelled with excitement and self-importance. I had made a major breakthrough. I had touched this man with my words and he had responded. I had discovered something truly important - Tam could communicate.

Using one squeeze for yes, two for no, I spent the morning deluging Tam with questions. Are you cold? Are you comfortable? Do you want another pillow? Poor Tam had no signal for go away and give me some peace. When not one more yes or no question would come to my mind, I finally released him. It was time to do my morning charting. I was a truly happy student nurse. My chest was inflated to the point of almost filling out my uniform. I began to eloquently chart how I had taught Tam the system of yes or no squeezes.

The importance of what I was charting gripped me. These were Tam's first recorded thoughts since the accident. I meticulously wrote down everything. Yes, he was cold; no, he did not want another pillow, on and on I went, filling up pages in the chart. No one would ever again pick up this chart without realizing Tam could express himself. This gave Tam the power to say yes or no, the power to make a decision regarding his life. I felt I had helped him regain some of his personal control and dignity.

All of this charting took a long time. I had just enough time to give Tam his noon feeding before taking my lunch break. I hurried back from my lunch to see what else I could discover and then chart about Tam. I entered his room to find his bed surrounded by friends and relatives. Six people circled his bed. The three older people sat in chairs quietly pensive. The three young people were in their early twenties like Tam. They were animated, talking rapidly in Chinese and English. I joined the group and introduced myself. I was tremendously excited to share my news with them. This could be one of those moments that brought everyone closer together.

My face was glowing hot my excitement was so intense. I had not imagined I would be the one that got to tell the family Tam can communicate. "Tam can talk," I was excited to explain, "look, he can squeeze his fingers once for yes, twice for no! You can talk to him, and he can talk back!"

One of the young women spoke first, "Yes, but we find it's much faster if he just blinks his eyes. If you look closely you can see the space between the tape, we can talk much faster this way. And we use two for yes, and one for no."

I looked at Tam and he blinked twice. They were tiny little quick blinks, as fast as if he had spoken the word. He didn't have the automatic blink response that keeps the eyes moist, but with a conscious effort, he could blink. All morning I had made him laboriously squeeze my hand, over and over. It was good physical therapy for him, but I felt like an idiot. I also felt cheated. Someone had climbed this mountain before me, and had done a much better job of it. The group didn't seem to notice the light going out of my face. They were happy to explain things to a staff member, no matter how lowly she may be. They told me what Tam liked and didn't like, and what he could and couldn't do.

It makes me think there should be a separate place for the families and loved ones to make notes. They could be handed chart sheets at the nursing station to use, and these could be added to the charts by the staff. Visitors are frequently aware of important things that the staff has not noticed. If I were a family member I would feel less impotent and more involved if I could write down along with the staff what I saw going on with the patient. Hospitals are too frightened to do this. Families might write something the hospital's legal staff would not want to hear.

The visitors left, Tam was ready to rest, and I went back to the charts. This was not as heady an experience as my first writing. I wrote down everything I had learned from the family and Tam. This made my earlier charting look pretty ridiculous. I would have loved to have ripped it out. But charts are legal documents, supposedly not to be tampered with. Avoiding looking like a Bozo student nurse didn't merit breaking the law.

Gilbert stayed up to date on the progress each of us was making with our patients. Over the next few days he marveled at my ability to perform psychosocial nursing on a semicomatose patient. I did all of the necessary physical stuff for Tam. I suctioned him every two hours, turned him regularly so he wouldn't get bed sores, and ran his meals down to his stomach through a tube. What I enjoyed most though was working with him and his family, discussing his progress, planning the direction of his care. We were all hopeful to get him into a rehabilitation center as soon as possible.

About the third day I worked with Tam, I had gone out of the room to get fresh linens to change his bed. When I returned something was wrong. Tam was struggling and gasping. I immediately checked his airway and found the respirator tube had come loose from his tracheotomy. Tam couldn't breathe. I reattached the tubing, gave him a couple of minutes to get some air, then suctioned him to make sure everything was fully patent. Once I finished, Tam began to quiet down and I broke out in quiet panic. What if I had stopped to use the bathroom or to chat with another nurse?

"God Tam, that scared me to death, you must have been terrified." Two blinks, yes, he was terrified. Silently dying of suffocation, within hearing distance of help, had to be the cruelest form of helplessness I could imagine. Something had to be done; the thought of losing Tam so senselessly was chilling. Throughout the morning as I worked, I searched for a solution. Tam's very limited vision made it impossible for him to see the cord attached to the light to alert the nurses that they were needed. Even if I attached it to his bed where he could always find it, he didn't have the dexterity to pull a string.

It was during my lunch break in my room that I came up with a solution. One of my friends had left a day-glow green tennis ball on my desk. I took the ball back to the ward with me. I grabbed some masking tape and taped the light cord to the ball so that it would never come off. I tied extra string to the cord so that it was long enough for the tennis ball to lie in bed inside the grasp of Tam's hand. I talked away at Tam the whole time, telling him my plan. I placed the ball in his hand and we began to practice. "Pull the ball as hard as you can." It wasn't easy for him; he worked for a half an hour before he learned to pull the ball down and turn on the light.

It was not a fail-safe solution. It was just the best I could come up with. Gilbert strolled by toward the end of our shift. I showed him my contraption, and Tam's new talent. I told him what necessitated the invention. "Well he's got to get off the respirator," Gilbert said in his British clip. "Rancho won't take him for rehabilitation if he's on a respirator." Rancho Los Amigos was the rehabilitation hospital to which County patients went; it had an excellent reputation. Gilbert said this as if it was no big deal. Tam just had to wean himself from the respirator.

"The doctors must know this" I said, "they must be going to do something." "Well they haven't done it yet, have they? No, its time this boy was off the respirator. We'll give it a try tomorrow. Then we can get him on his way to Rancho, be much better for him there." Then Gilbert turned his broad backside to me, and walked away. Just like that, we were going to wean Tam off his respirator. No doctors orders, no huge consultations, no debates. Just Gilbert and me, saying give it a try, it's time the boy should be moving on, and getting better.

Gilbert showed up by my side early the next morning. "Here we go, no problem," he said. I was slightly terrified. I wasn't sure what we were doing was even legal. When I get scared and totally unsure, I think about the legalities of things. Instead of seeing boogie men, I see lawyers and lawsuits. This makes sense; lawyers and law codes are sort of the modern day version of the boogie man. Gilbert was obviously not thinking about the law, so I figured he was not afraid. He probably knew what he was doing.

Gilbert explained it to Tam. "I am going to remove the respirator tube, and you must try to breathe." Nothing very sophisticated or tricky about that, I thought, I was still timid, though. I was concerned some type of alarm would sound the minute an illicit nursing procedure was performed. Gilbert removed the respirator tube and said "breathe Tam, breathe Tam." He gave Tam some time to try, and then gave him a few minutes of air, before trying again.

"Breathe Tam, breathe Tam," this time my voice joined Gilbert's. Five minutes of this was enough work for the moment. "Not bad," Gilbert said, "I think he'll get it. We'll give it another try tomorrow." Gilbert left and I talked to Tam about how much better it would be for him if he could make it to Rancho. After a while, his family and friends arrived. I told them what we were doing, the plan we had in mind. I told Tam's doctor too, who looked at me with doubt. He stood there with two other doctors listening to me as if I were a child. I wouldn't drop the subject, so the doctor disconnected Tam's respirator for a moment and said, "see, he can't breathe". He reconnected Tam and walked off.

The family reacted to the concept differently. If Tam needed to breathe before he could move on, Tam would learn to breath. They began to work with him aggressively. Family visits were no longer social encounters but training sessions. With no official permission, or doctor's orders, the family would remove Tam's air supply and demand he breathe. I stood back far enough not to be involved, but close enough to watch and be there if I was needed. It seemed to me they were making progress.

I had been off the unit for the weekend. When I returned on Monday morning I already knew my assignment, and went straight to Tam's room. I was surprised to find much of the family gathered around him. My anxiety rose, I went over to see what was going on. A stretcher on wheels was pushed in front of me before I reached Tam's bed.

"He's on his way, he's going to Rancho, thanks for your help." The whole group of them pushed right on out the door, with Tam on a stretcher in the center of them. I never really got a look at his face. There was no chance to say anything. I stood there looking at his empty bed, with the call light still attached to the bright green tennis ball. Beside the bed, the unneeded respirator stood silent. I suddenly felt empty and discarded, which was an unreasonable way to feel when something so right had just happened.

It had happened without me, because I was only one of the small players, not a central character. But Tam had been central to me. He had held my focus and my heart for two weeks, and now he was gone. People don't know this about nurses. They don't know about how we have to let go. They assume it is our job. It is our job to care. But we only are assumed to care for as long as we are needed. The partings are abrupt. No one speaks of the emotional attachments that can take place.

No one assumed a student nurse on the day shift would have any strong feelings about a patient being transferred. I kept my hurt inside and gave no one any indication that they should think differently. I missed getting to say good-bye to Tam. I missed even more getting to celebrate with him. I missed having a moment of shared joy, just to say you made it, you are on your way, and receiving two blinks in response.

A new patient was in the bed across from Tam's vacated one. He was a young man, powerfully built, and thrashing around in his bed. His arms and legs were tied to the bed, to prevent him from doing too much damage to himself with the thrashing. He was constantly emitting soft moans and groans. His incessant movement prevented the staff from being able to keep his body covered. A sheet had been woven around his waist and between his legs to prevent exposing his genitals, but otherwise he was naked. He was in great shape. Muscles rippled everywhere under tan skin as he twisted and torqued his arms and legs. His hair had been shaved to within an eighth of an inch from his scalp, to expose his head wounds for cleaning.

I found him frightening from the perspective of having to work with him. It was also intimidating to think how easily this could happen. I read his chart and realized he had rolled his Jeep in the hills. A day of fun in the sun had come to a dire end. This boy was much more distressing to me than Tam had been. Tam had lain there quietly, almost as if at peace. This boy was a wild thing, all turmoil and agitation.

I asked one of the nurses, "How bad is he?" "He's a lucky one", she said, "he's only got a minor head injury. He should clear up in a while. He'll be alright then, there's nothing else wrong with him." This was a whole different perspective on what indicated a minor or a major head injury than what I had learned in nursing school. The boy's name was Tommy, and I took a closer look at him to see if I could discern what the nurse was talking about.

Once I got past his wild appearance, I notice he didn't have as many tubes in him as most of the other patients. Tommy was able to breathe on his own. He didn't need a respirator or extra oxygen to help him out. That's how he was able to produce so much noise. He had no IV, just a nasogastric tube for feeding him. The catheter he wore was an external one, which meant they didn't think he would be needing it long, or they would have inserted an indwelling one. Then again, they may have been afraid that all his thrashing would displace an internal one, and cause him injury. He looked like a healthy young male, who just wasn't conscious.

Gilbert came in and gave me the news that Tommy was my next patient. I groaned, there was not going to be any communication with this young man. Tommy was really out of it. He was also big, which meant he would provide plenty of hard physical work for me. The good news was that without a respirator I was spared from suctioning. I took a few minutes to read through Tommy's chart more carefully. It only took a few minutes because he had just been admitted last night.

There wasn't much information. Tommy had been driving his jeep in the Hollywood hills. Somehow he had lost control and rolled the jeep over the side of a hill. His body had some minor cuts and scrapes. The only real injury was to his head. There was no indication of permanent brain damage, but they would have to wait until he regained consciousness to assess what was intact and what wasn't. The current guarded opinion was that Tommy would come through this pretty well. This did not rule out the highly probable need for intensive rehabilitation therapy once he was conscious and stable.

With that little bit of information I set out to do my morning chores taking care of Tommy. Gilbert gave me the good news that since we were familiar with the unit now, and my current patient was such a breeze, he was also assigning me two more. I was given another man and a woman. They were two of the sickest patients I had ever had. Both were fully tubed, on respirators, and not expected to live long.

The man was listed as "NO CODE." This is an unofficial classification that means do not resuscitate. If his heart stopped beating I was to leave him peacefully alone and notify the nursing station. Both of these patients were in their eighties and totally unconscious. The man especially had trouble breathing, even with a respirator. I was always afraid he would die while I was suctioning him. I was very lucky. In my several years in nursing I never experienced the death of a patient. While working with these patients I had constant concern that I might accidentally push one of them over the edge.

The most memorable aspect of taking care of Tommy was getting to know his mother and his roommate Mark. At noon on the first day I took care of Tommy, Mark showed up at his bedside. I walked in on a one-sided conversation, with Mark updating Tommy on all the events of the last twenty-four hours. Tommy thrashed and softly groaned, while Mark chatted away like this was normal procedure. He had brought a stack of books and was debating out loud which one he thought Tommy would like to hear him read.

Mark was a slightly built man, with a soft blond look, which was very different from Tommy's swarthy robust appearance. Mark had the look and intensity of a serious student. Observing the concern on his face, and the warmth in his eyes, it was clear to me these young men were lovers, and not just in the sense of just having sex with one another. In light of that, it seemed only appropriate for me to interact with Mark as I would any visiting spouse. We talked about their lives together, and their plans for the future. I told Mark that a fine rehabilitation center was not too far from where they lived. Mark and Tommy were young and struggling to get by on very little money while they were in school. The thought of Tommy getting good care close to their home was reassuring.

Late the next morning Mark was reading aloud to Tommy when Tommy's mother arrived. She was an impeccably groomed, conservatively dressed Boston matron in her late-forties. She was chilly and stiff, here to take charge of her son's care. While her outer layer yelled confident and competent, her inner layer seemed frightened and unsure. She had flown in a rush from the East coast to see her son who had been injured. She found him in a county hospital, tied to a bed, with another young man encamped in a chair next to him. Tough news to get dumped on a mother all at once.

Mark introduced himself as Tommy's roommate. Mrs. Robinson's instincts seemed to tell her immediately what the situation was. I was again playing the social hostess, trying to make a place for each person to feel comfortable while Tommy thrashed around on the bed in front of us. A mother had almost lost her son, a lover had almost lost his love, and neither were able to pull themselves away from his bedside. I had to go on with my work. I still needed to bathe Tommy, change his linens, and feed him his lunch. I decided it was best to proceed and make it a family event.

Mrs. Robinson was the newest on the scene, and the least at ease. Tommy's large, muscular, nearly naked body lay between the three of us. We each had our own form of intimacy with this unconscious young man. Mrs. Robinson had met his physical needs as a child. Mark had been the one to hold Tommy as an adult. Now that he was returned to a state of infantile neediness, I was the one to take care of him. We were a daisy chain of caretakers.

I knew the rules. I was supposed to ask the visitors to leave, pull the drapes and give Tommy his bed bath. It seemed unfair and cruel to me. These were the people who loved him, and had a need to care for him, but it was my job. I gathered the hot water, towels, wash clothes, and drew the drapes enclosing the four of us. The wash clothes were handed out. We each took a body part and began to clean. I was working on his legs, Mark took his chest and arms, and Mrs. Robinson was carefully cleaning Tommy's face.

She was still a little nervous with the whole thing - her son's coma, a county hospital, and the idea of Mark. Mrs. Robinson covered her nerves with mindless chatter. "This is really a very nice hospital Tommy. The people are so pleasant. You are a very lucky boy to have such a pretty nurse Tommy. Can you see your pretty nurse." Mark's eye caught mine and we smiled. Mrs. Robinson saw the smile, and it turned into a giggle. She blushed, looked back into her son's face, and then she just sort of released. Her careful posture softened, her face looked sad instead of tense, and the mindless chatter stopped.

The bath proceeded quietly, each person being with Tommy in their own way. We took turns dipping into the hot water and ringing out our wash clothes. We handed soap and towels back and forth. There was some talk, but it was soft, and as likely to be directed to one another as to Tommy. We talked about how he looked to us. Tommy was there as a silent fourth. We told him what we saw.

I had started cleaning at his feet, worked my way up his legs, until finally I was at the sheet covering Tommy's groin. I hadn't thought this far ahead. I paused, staring at that last bit of sheet, thinking what am I going to do now? Bed baths on comatose patients are not too tricky, you just clean their genitals. If there is a catheter you make sure everything is intact, and working fine. But I stalled. I wasn't ready to confront Tommy's genitals, particularly with his mother and lover together for the first time.

I looked up directly into the eyes of Mark and Mrs. Robinson, who seemed to sense my dilemma. "I have to check, to make sure everything is OK here." And then I just waited to see what they would do. They smiled sympathetically, and waited, looking concerned. They wanted to know if everything was OK there too. So that was it, the four of us were in this together. I was currently breaking several hospital rules. I lifted up the sheet to take a peek. Mark's and Mrs. Robinson's heads craned to take a peek with me. We took a look, let out a collective sigh, and looked up with disappointed eyes to console each other. The catheter had come off and the sheets were soaked.

I was now in a situation in which I truly did not want to be. I couldn't cut these people out now just because the going got tough. I had made a silent pact with them to let them stay. I told them "I have to go and get another catheter set up." I figured this gave them the perfect opportunity to leave if they wanted. Tommy's mother had more grit than I had realized. She said "Fine, we will take care of washing him up while you do that. Then the three of us can change his sheets." I turned to go, leaving Mark and Mrs. Robinson pressed head to head over Tommy's genitals.

I figured luckily Gilbert was a creative thinker. If he walked in and found mother and lover working away at their task, he might see the humor or at least the humanity in it. Hopefully, I wouldn't be kicked out of school. I returned to the undisturbed curtains and slipped inside. I was greeted by a nice, clean, dry penis, and a smiling, proud Mark and Mrs. Robinson. I didn't even ask how this was accomplished. I was just grateful. We changed his sheets, and then I began setting about to reapply the condom catheter.

Tommy's penis was long and thick and very soft, the worst possible thing in the world to try and secure in a condom catheter. I would have felt awkward in front of Tommy's mother. I would have felt awkward in front of his lover. Together, the three of us stared at the task that lay ahead of me. I began to speak, and that seemed to help things out. "I need to roll this condom on over his penis." I was stalling, hoping someone would come up with a thought.

Mark was able to make some sense of things. "I will hold him upright like this, and then you can have two hands to work the condom down." Mrs. Robinson was not to be left out, "I'll cut some tape so it will be ready for you." We began. Mark and I had the toughest job; jello would have been easier to corral. By the time the condom was fully in place, Mrs. Robinson had managed to cut more than twenty pieces of tape. I hated letting her know I only needed one.

Eventually my chores were done, Tommy was fed, and I was drained. Working via committee is much more difficult than working solo. Mark and Mrs. Robinson didn't look at all drained. They looked relaxed, and even happy. They had settled into chairs. Mark was beginning to read to the two of them. I told them both good-bye, and took off for my dorm room to lunch in solitude, just me and **Bewitched.**

I worked with Tommy for just one week before my rotation on Neurological Medicine came to an end. Every day Mark and Mrs. Robinson were there at his bedside. They continued to stay involved and were a great deal of help to me in taking care of him. However, I made sure to get the intimate chores out of the way before any visitors arrived. I figured I was lucky, I hadn't gotten caught and thrown out of school. Probably Gilbert would have just lectured me on a patient's right to privacy and made me feel like an idiot.

Mrs. Robinson was strongly considering taking Tommy to a rehabilitation center back East. She wanted him to be near her, and she was sure facilities would be better on the East coast. Mark was in a terrible, powerless position. She was the blood relative, she had the right to make the decision. Gilbert and I talked to her about her options. We sang the praises of Rancho Los Amigos rehabilitation hospital. We talked about the importance of the support of his friends during Tommy's recuperation. Mark and Tommy seemed especially close. It would be almost impossible for them to be together if Tommy was taken East.

Things were talked about in careful, delicate language. Friend and roommate were substituted for lover and mate. Mrs. Robinson was not deceived, but she was not forced to acknowledge something publicly before she was ready. I had only one day left on the wards and Gilbert poured on the steam. He talked about the closeness of the boys, their need to be together. I think the depth of Mark's love and concern was what won her over in the end. Gilbert's and my arguments only gave rational form to her heart's leanings. The decision was made. Tommy would go to Rancho as soon as he was ready. Mrs. Robinson would fly back and visit him as often as she could. Mark offered to let her stay at his and Tommy's place, but she looked a little green at the thought.

Gilbert knew I was truly happy. It would have really bothered me to see these men separated. He had probably interfered more than he would have on Mark's behalf, because he knew I wanted it so badly. Our senior instructors gave us each an evaluation at this point before we went on to team leading. I sat in Gilbert's office tensed to hear his assessment of my skills and abilities. "You are a competent nurse. You are not Intensive Care quality, but I have no complaints about your skills. You deserve to graduate. What you are is a psych nurse. That's all there is to it. It's where you belong."

I didn't mind the Psychiatric part, that's where I was planning to go. But I wasn't thrilled about the competent part. Gilbert had judged my skills pretty much the way I did. I was a technically competent nurse. I had sort of hoped that somehow I was mistaken, that actually I was a technically magnificent nurse. I was secretly hoping that Gilbert had discovered this, and I was eager to receive his accolades. Instead I was told what I already knew. I belonged on psych.

Being a technically competent nurse was hard work for me. My stomach constantly churned, my head grew light, and I have required assistance from fellow students to exit a few hospital rooms while still on my feet. Gilbert may have known the inner battle I faced every time the goo began to flow. In light of this, I was able to take some pride in myself for having become a competent nurse. I never thought I had the stuff to do it. I wasn't going to have to do it much longer though, because I was going on to do psychiatric nursing on 6-A when I graduated.

Our evaluation meeting with Gilbert was also the time when we were to make our decision on where we wanted to do our team leading. I had the choice of Infected Ortho or Neuro Med. It wasn't a difficult decision for me. I needed patients I could talk to, even if I occasionally pissed them off. I also wanted the wise and sympathetic tutelage of Cheryl South, the head nurse on Infected Orthopedics. So it was back to the pus unit for my last few weeks as a student nurse at County.

Chapter Twenty-Six

After Hours

Mrs. Sherman, the head nurse of the adolescent psych unit, was a very persuasive person. During the last two weeks of my psychiatric rotation she convinced me that not only did I belong there permanently as a staff member when I graduated, but that I should begin working there part-time, evenings, now. I am a good hard worker, when I need to work. When I don't need to work, I would rather not. I had just enough money to get through school without working. I didn't really want to take on an evening job. I would rather read a good book or watch even an average movie than go to work if I don't really need the money to survive. I would rather shop the discount stores and skip the specialty shops than work extra hours unnecessarily.

I didn't think this was a wise thing to explain to my future boss. I generally like my bosses to think of me as eager. I wanted to appear eager to work with the kids, eager to be on the unit, and even eager for the money. 6A was a plum of a job, if you like psych, which I did. I didn't want to blow it by telling Annie Sherman that I really didn't want to work unless it was a necessity. Annie could lean on you with guilt, and ooze on you with charm, all at the same time. After two years of working with her, I only improved a little at telling Annie, "no." Most people never got that far.

By the last six months of nursing school, most of my friends were working three or more eight hour shifts a week. Evelyn and Susan both worked several nights a week from three to eleven p.m. Senior students frequently worked on the units that they would eventually go to work on full time. This works out great for County. There is no time lost training new nurses. By the time students graduate and start work they know what they are doing. Listening to my friends talk, I could tell they had become comfortable with the hospital and the duties required of an R.N.

I hadn't made that transition yet. Three months from graduation, and I was still afraid of how I would function as an R.N. responsible for a unit of patients and staff. I knew I wouldn't be responsible for everything at the beginning, but eventually it would come. On the psych unit I wouldn't have long to wait. There was only one R.N. assigned to a unit on weekends, and he or she was responsible for the eighteen patients, staff, and whatever chaos arose. I figured that money aside, I better get my butt over there and leaR.N. what was going on while I was still a student. It's much better to make a multitude of mistakes as a student than it is as a full-time staff member.

Eleven p.m. is just too late to work. I am nearly in a sleep coma by ten. I saw no reason why I couldn't get the experience I needed between the hours of five and nine p.m. I didn't want to go over at three, because I needed some time after wards and classes to relax and have some dinner. None of my friends worked this schedule. They were all hardy and worked full eight hour shifts. I explained to Annie that I needed time to study, always a valid student excuse. It also seemed like I wasn't really needed on the unit once the kids went to bed at nine. Annie was willing to work with me. Throughout the years I worked for her, she remained flexible, and I maintained a creative schedule.

My previous experience with 6A had consisted of three days a week, moR.N.ings until noon. Most of this early moR.N.ing tIme is very structured for the kids. Getting dressed and having breakfast goes on until eight-thirty when everyone gathers in the dayroom for group. From nine-thirty until ten or ten-thirty, the doctors and staff held rounds. Patients had private sessions with their doctors, family meetings, and sessions with the recreational therapist or the school teacher until noon, when lunch was served. By one o'clock everyone was in bed for a nap. I may have seen a little bit of havoc and craziness as a student nurse, but it wasn't until I started working evenings that I really got a sense of 6A.

I had not yet met any of the evening staff. The person to whom I reported was the charge nurse on evenings, Leona Walker. No one ever called her anything but Walker. Just like in the military, no first name, no Ms. This fit her perfectly. She had a sturdy body, short black hair, olive skin, pretty dark brown eyes enlarged by thick glasses, and a large beautiful white smile. The smile was not a permanent fixture. It came out rarely, like the sun in Coastal Oregon, and was just as refreshing. Her clothing was always sensible, her manner frequently abrupt. Much like myself, when working, she had a very serious air about her. I think Walker was a couple of years younger than myself. Her demeanor and appearance seemed ten years older. She nursed like a veteran, practical, functional, no excessive softness, or unnecessary concern. I experienced my immediate superior as cold, exacting, and intimidating. I did not want to screw up in front of Walker.

I also saw Walker as cold and hard with the kids. Over time, I realized she was someone they trusted, a rock of sanity in a sea of turbulent emotions. When the kids needed her she was there. Later, when I began working full-time on days, there were several times when Walker showed up on her off-duty time to lend a child emotional support during a difficult family meeting.

Walker introduced me to the evening staff. There was one other R.N., Miss Lightly. Miss Lightly was a tiny bird of an Australian woman. She was extremely conscientious and followed every rule in the book, making her a target for the antics of the staff and kids. Miss Lightly also sold Amway products on the side. I can still see her demonstrating a drain cleaner, "So safe you can drink it." After a display like that I had to buy some, even if I didn't have a drain.

There were usually four attendants working evenings, two men, and two women. They were a streetwise clique. I always felt naive and very sheltered around these people. 6A was about the only thing our lives held in common. I was considered a college girl from the suburbs, just floating through, nothing to take too seriously. I felt like Alice slipping down the rabbit hole each evening as I stepped across the locked threshold of 6A. I would thrust my key in the lock, tuR.N. it, and enter into the unpredictability of the evening.

I began getting a sense of myself here by playing with the patients. I would involve myself in games as soon as possible. I played checkers, Ping-Pong, pool, and Pente. I can be shy and not very outgoing. I was grateful to any individual who would come up and ask me to play with them. This is how I began to get to know the kids and staff of 6A. I would play games and we would talk. This is also how I came to know Cathy, a sixteen year old frequent visitor to 6A.

Cathy told me this had been her third suicide attempt. She always used pills, because it was the only method she could stand. Cathy was five feet four inches tall, overweight, with limp blond hair. Her eyes were blue, her smile was rare, and her breasts were large. She had the potential to be pretty. She told me she had been pretty, when she was young. At thirteen and fourteen she had a great figure. Now she was just old and fat. She said it was just as well, her stepfather wasn't nearly as interested in her now that she was fat. She thought this probably made her mother feel better.

Cathy was the first of many teenage girls to become my "daughters." They were always very bright, with a sense of humor, and entrenched in a life painful beyond all reason. I played with lots of kids every evening, but Cathy's face was the one I sought out and attempted to read first. The bond always goes two ways. My presence made Cathy smile; she felt she had a priority on my affections, and she did.

It is the doctor's job, to stay clinical and not get emotionally involved. Thankfully the nursing staff is given the freedom to care deeply about their patients. This can be complicated, but there is balance here, for where there is affection there is also dislike. My pet was someone else's bane and vice versa. Where I might see only Cathy's pain and intense need for love and self-acceptance, others saw a pain in the butt, or a manipulative and moody girl. Both sides were true, both needed to be addressed. The enamored staff member was usually the one to talk with the patient and sort out emotional and behavioral issues. "Go find out what the hell is the matter with your daughter today, she is in a terrible mood." The disenchanted staff member kept one from being too blind and losing one's perspective.

Cathy was no angel. She told me one evening that she had been planing to elope the evening before. Eloping is a euphemism for escaping. Her plan was to follow me out to the door. She would talk and joke and keep me company as I left. She figured I would assume she was tagging along to tell me good-bye, and she was right. I trusted Cathy. I had opened my heart to care for her, and I expected her to be straight with me. This is a great deal to expect of a sixteen-year-old in a locked psychiatric facility who has attempted suicide three times. I was extremely naive, a disease I never completely conquered in my two years on 6A.

I was so naive that Cathy couldn't do it. It was too easy. She couldn't be the one to turn the light on for me, to show me the real world where people will use other people, even ones they like. She told me about her plan, and then she became angry with me. "You should be more careful, you could get hurt that way. I was going to push you aside to get out of the door. Me or somebody else may want to get out, so you have to be more careful." She complained to me, "I couldn't go, because I knew if I did you would feel bad, and take it personally." She was right. I would have felt hurt and abandoned. I would have taken it personally. So she stayed.

At sixteen, Cathy had lived a hundred more years than I had. Maybe what drew her to me was my innocence and my belief in the innate goodness of people, which was something she had lost at puberty. Some of my most striking early lessons in Psychiatry involved Cathy. I am certain she added much more to my growing up process than I ever added to her's.

We were sitting on the couch one evening, and three or four of the kids were making comments about the news. Six o'clock medications had been passed out an hour earlier and everyone was settling down for the evening. I noticed an absence of caustic remarks from Cathy regarding Lady Di's reported virginity, so I looked over at her. Her head was twisted back at a strange angle. She was starting to grimace and make an odd face. I became conceR.N.ed and began questioning her. "Cathy, what's the matter? Talk to me! Why are you holding your head like that, can you move it?"

A fourteen-year-old girl interrupted my barrage of questions and suggested that Cathy needed the nurse. I recognized a sane comment, and immediately went for Walker. With a minimal amount of coherency I blurted out, "Cathy is sitting with her head all funny and can't talk."

Walker stayed calm and quiet in her attitude, while she moved quickly. "She's having EPS." With no other explanation it was expected that I would understand. She left for the dayroom and Cathy's side. I trailed behind Walker watching every move she made, while wracking my brain trying to remember what EPS was. She reached Cathy and put her arm around her shoulder. "Cathy, it's Walker. I am going to give you some medication to take care of that." With her arm around the teenager to control her body, in one smooth move Walker had Cathy on her feet and walking to a bed in an isolation room.

I was told to stay with Cathy while Walker went for the medication. I felt truly useless sitting there, trying to be of comfort. Cathy, Walker, the rest of the kids and staff on the unit, everyone knew what was going on but me. While I sat in angst on Cathy's bed, her head torqued farther and farther to the back and the side. Her eyes rolled up to the top of her head. She couldn't speak at all. A lifetime later, Walker finally arrived with a loaded syringe. She found a nice meaty spot, and sent the medication in. Then she sat on the opposite side of the bed from me. She spoke softly with Cathy, and waited.

In about fifteen minutes Cathy's symptoms started to clear up. Walker talked to her a little more, and then left me to stay while she did the paper work. Once Cathy was able to speak the first thing I asked her was, "Cathy, why didn't you tell me you needed help?" If I ever have EPS I hope the last thing I have to deal with on coming out of it is an anxious student nurse. Now, as I consider her situation, I think Cathy was extremely patient with me. She said, "You kept asking me questions, but I couldn't talk." The nice thing is, she didn't call me an idiot, or a jerk, or any of the equally appropriate terms she could have used.

Cathy and other patients continued to experience EPS symptoms intermittently during the time I worked on 6A. After that first time, I went home and did my reading. EPS stands for extra pyramidal symptoms, one of the most common side effects of almost all anti-psychotic drugs. According to my 1980 Goodman and Gilman's ***The Pharmacological Basis of Therapeutics***, Sixth Edition, the mechanism for these drugs affecting the extrapyramidal part of the nervous system is not yet known. Cathy's symptoms were the classic side effects seen when beginning anti-psychotic medication treatment. The reaction is called acute dystonia, which means she had spasms of the tongue, face, neck, and back. The spasms cause facial grimacing, a twisted neck, and her eyes to roll up until the iris can barely be seen. The combined effect can mimic a seizure, so you have to know your patient's meds and assess them carefully. There are other types of extra-pyramidal symptoms associated with prolonged use of anti-psychotics, but our patients were here for short stays, so Cathy's was the type we saw frequently.

One of the main things Cathy was there to teach me about was my limitations, and she was a relentless teacher. I had been on the unit several weeks and was feeling pretty good about my ability to talk with the patients. I might even have been bordering on the smug. The luck of the beginner had made me swell with feelings of power and confidence. I was even beginning to feel my touch for this might be better than Walker's. I might have a gift for this. As my competitive spirit reared its head, I should have known I was in for trouble. But as I recognize it only rarely now, the chances of my having seen it then are nil.

The trouble took about a week to find me. It was around seven o'clock one evening and I was deeply engrossed in a card game with Cathy. We had been talking the whole time and the conversation had tuR.N.ed very serious. She had begun to talk about her step-father and their relationship. I had read her whole chart and hadn't seen anything special about him in there. Up until now she had only made references to me about his liking to look at her in her bikini. I thought this conversation was important. She needed to talk about this relationship and I could be a supportive listener.

I listened while Cathy poured out her feelings about her step-father molesting her at thirteen and raping her at fourteen. I had never heard something like this first-hand before. I stayed with her, listening, reassuring her that it wasn't her fault. I did all that I could figure out to do. But I didn't go get Walker and say, "Cathy is talking about some very painful stuff, and I am probably in over my head in dealing with it." I think my feelings of empathy for Cathy were so overwhelming, I didn't think about what would be most helpful to her. I am sorry to think that my competitive spirit with Walker may also have inhibited me from seeking her help.

I muddled along until finally Cathy was overloaded with pain. She said she needed some time alone. I nodded that I understood, and let her go seek some peace and privacy. I had no idea of the depth of the pain that she was dealing with. In my naiveté I assumed she was probably having a private moment to cry in solitude and to collect herself. I thought she would feel better now that she had talked about it.

I had loosened a cork on a tightly sealed bottle, one that had been sitting on the shelf fermenting for years. I found her twenty minutes later curled up into a ball on the floor in the hallway, behind an open door. I sat on the floor with her, wrapped my arms around her, and tried to be of comfort. Caring for Cathy as much as I did, her pain was terrible for me. My fury at her step-father was intense and blinding.

The close contact was too much for her; she needed to move. I walked her to her bedroom where we both sat on her bed. County has very few spare chairs. Cathy had stopped crying and had become tense and quiet. I never knew what happened next. Suddenly she was on me. She outweighed me by at least fifty pounds, and she was blind with rage. My shock and confusion were intense. She had me on the floor before I could scream for Walker. When I did finally yell it must have been loud because Walker was there very quickly. I hadn't had time to understand what was happening, when I realized the three of us were wrestling with all our strength on the floor.

Cathy struggled to inflict all of her pain outward, while Walker and I fought to restrain her without anyone being injured. Walker was an expert at this, and after a few moments Cathy was pinned safely with her back to the floor. I grabbed a pillow to protect the back of her head, while Walker yelled, "Code Three, Code Three!"

Cathy taught me first-hand the meaning of "Code Three." There was yelling in the halls, and the sounds of attendants running towards us. Someone had called the code into the central nursing station downstairs. The p.a. system was announcing, "Code Three, 6A; Code Three, 6A." The two male attendants arrived first, and replaced Walker in holding Cathy down. I stayed in place, holding the pillow under her head and talking to her. Walker left for the medication room. Finally, a female attendant arrived with leather restraints for Cathy's wrists and ankles. The front door to the unit banged open and four large male attendants came rushing in. They were full of adrenaline, ready to throw themselves into the fray.

Walker had been very quick, and was already back with a loaded syringe. Cathy was expertly rolled onto her side and a two inch square of skin was exposed on her left hip. No checking for landmarks, the needle was in and out in a flash. Two more male attendants pushed through the door, but they knew they were slow to respond and had probably missed all of the good stuff. Cathy had quieted now and was only crying. We carefully lifted her onto the bed, and the attendants affixed the restraints to her bed. The job was done, the show was over. The men nodded, satisfied that everything was under control. Everybody filed out of the room. I stayed with Cathy to talk with her and rub her head until she fell asleep. With a hundred milligrams of Thorazine on board, it didn't take long.

I sat on Cathy's bed feeling completely shell-shocked. My body was shaking, and I began to cry. As she relaxed and became quiet, I slowly disintegrated. My heart was breaking, my mind was terrified; I thought this was my fault. I had hurt Cathy and she might have seriously hurt me. The immensity of the experience overwhelmed me. Cathy consoled me. She apologized for hurting me. She said this is what happens when she just gets so mad she can't take it anymore. Her tendeR.N.ess towards my anguish was the most loving thing she could have given me. She told me, "I feel much better with the restraints on, much safer. I'm gonna go to sleep now." I kissed her good night on the forehead, and sat there a while, collecting myself.

I pulled myself together and went in to face Walker. I must have looked just as terrified and broken-hearted as I felt. She handled me very gently. I explained what Cathy and I had been talking about, what I thought had caused her to "go off." During my two years on 6A, I became very familiar with kids "going off." But the first time was an explosion of mind and emotion that had left me completely shaken. Walker confirmed that a better way to handle the situation would have been to consult her very early in our discussion, and if not then, at any point sooner than I did.

She understood the lesson I had received was far beyond any she could give me. Walker was kind in pointing out that this was not an infrequent occurrence for Cathy. I was beginning to understand the depths of the pain some of these teenagers were experiencing. I learned to tread with care, as the footing was incredibly shaky. Later on I would also come to learn the importance of "going off" and the tremendous release of anger and pain a person can experience by a huge explosion of striking out. The attendants and the restraints were there to help prevent injuries to the staff and the patients. "Going off" or "blowing up" provided a way for a patient to release tremendous amounts of rage without having disastrous consequences. Many times, it was the only thing that would allow the healing to begin. Sometimes it was planned. The staff would prepare for the outburst, and then push the kid until it came. Dr. Blade, or Mrs. Sherman would say, "That kid needs to blow, and today is the day we're going to do it."

Tonight I had gotten my feet very wet. I had seen my first Code Three, with my favorite patient and myself at the center of it. It was ten-thirty before I left the unit, and walked across the street to my dorm. My legs had finally stopped shaking. I was drained to the point of feeling numb and hollow. This was the type of evening when it was nice to get back and find my roommate's connecting door open. I knocked and entered at the same time, holding a bottle of cheap burgundy in my hand. Susan got glasses, I poured, we talked.

None of us had the exact same experiences; no two people do. For the most part those of us muddling through County together spared each other our most private pain. I assume this because no one talked to me about the really difficult moments, the private times of searing, white-hot pain. Michael is the only one that occasionally shared these moments with me. But they came for me and I have to believe they came for others. What we did share was the unwinding. One didn't need to speak to what was the source of the need to unwind. There was a universal thread weaving through all of our experiences.

We talked about the units constantly. We talked about the insanity, the unbelievable state of chaos a body could be in, and still function. We marveled at the amazing adaptability of the mind and body. We dissected the hospital from every perspective - social, political, economic, medical, and nursing. We covered every topic in detail, except the emotional toll it could take on us.

We did not choose to incorporate self-disclosure into our coping mechanisms. We preferred escapism. There was Coors, Gallo, pot, humor, parties, sarcasm, sex, dates with doctors; take your pick. We did. I mostly chose a glass of wine and the company of Evelyn and Susan. I also chose movies and shopping, which were costly but excellent modes of escapism. My wardrobe flourished while I tucked away small painful moments.

Chapter Twenty-Seven

Rites Of Passage

There were many rites of passage for a student nurse at County, rites that reach back almost to the days of Florence herself. They are also almost extinct now. During my stint at County, the rites began the moment you signed on the dotted line.

It began even before the first day, when I went to the official uniform company to be fitted for my ill-fitting uniform. This was a private ceremony shared only with a lady with pins in her mouth. But I knew I was one of hundreds who had stood in this gray dressing room sweating and being stuck with pins wondering, "Why am I doing this?" I was doing it because it is the first ritual in which everyone participates as they find their way through the maze of acquiring a diploma in nursing from County.

After buying the uniform came the first day of school, followed months later by capping. Once we had our caps, from then on at the end of each term we were given a perpendicular stripe in black velvet. This was a hash mark to put on our cap indicating our progress and seniority in nursing school. The final capping rite came at graduation, when we would get a new cap with a single velvet stripe following the brim all the way around, indicating we were graduate nurses.

All of the time we would spend in school had been marked out for us. Exactly halfway through our experience came the Halfway Dinner. This was a semi-formal affair in a rented ballroom, sort of like a junior prom. A junior prom is just not something that cool antiestablishment types can go to and remain cool. A coat and tie made Gregory, Kevin, and the other cool guys turn green. The dinner dance was just too bourgeois for most of my friends. Therefore, I have no idea what the Halfway Dinner was like. Judging from the pictures of it in the annual, I would say I probably didn't miss much.

What I attended instead was an Alternative Halfway Dinner (by invitation only). A select group of about fifteen of us took part in a private dinner bash. Lee, Gregory's suite mate, was a magnificent gourmet cook. Lee's lover, Keith, had a home in South Pasadena that he kindly agreed to donate for our affair. The list included Evelyn, Susan and me, Annie Whammie, her best friend Cathleen, Sharon, Gregory, John, Kevin, and miscellaneous others. Kevin was the group stud that many of the girls either had, or dreamed of having before their time in nursing school was over. Gregory had been in an auto accident recently and had to attend with his jaw wired shut. Lee couldn't stand the thought of Gregory missing the taste of his beautiful food. Each dish was run through the blender so Gregory could sip the mush through a straw. I remember an evening of eating wonderful delicacies while watching Gregory suck green goo.

The next major marker after Halfway Dinner was One Hundred Days. Which meant there were one hundred days left until we were all through on the wards. It had nothing to do with classes or finals. Just one hundred days left until we could burn those God-awful uniforms. This was a major event. The seniors on each floor devised a plan to decorate their floors in a ritual competition. The decorations were to be installed on the day of, and judged the evening of, One Hundred Days.

I am not a planner, plotter, or joiner of group activities. Eager beaver has never been an adjective applied to me. This is why I was on the periphery of the cool group; I am a periphery person. The complexity of the decorations that were required for this event called for the serious leaders to man the helm. On each floor there was a room designated for the planners and designers to gather. These were usually the younger girls in their very early twenties, and some of the more involved older ones.

I would look in on these meetings. The girls were dressed in pajamas and sweats, their bodies spilling over all of the furniture and floor space. I would see buddies, with their arms and legs draped over each other, and a huge bowl of popcorn or dip in the middle of the floor. The women's floors of the dorm constantly had the feel of a pajama party. This feeling was intensified during the complex preparations for One Hundred Days.

I was never invited to help plan. Susan and I must have seemed somewhat foreign to these young women. They didn't picture us as the types to get excited about decorations. Maybe they thought we sat around having political and philosophical discussions all the time. I guess that sounds boring, but its pretty accurate, except when we were curled up watching "Little House on the Prairie." A few days before the Big Day, a young woman approached Susan and me, and asked if we would like to help with the decorations. "Yes," we wanted to do that, it sounded like fun. We didn't want to miss out on the experience completely. We were given a very mundane task that we couldn't possibly screw up. We were supposed to cut flowers out of pink and lavender paper. I think they figured that if we weren't seriously dedicated to this, they didn't want to tax our enthusiasm. I think their decision showed wisdom. Susan and I managed to do our small part adequately, and to finish it before we became bored.

I had no idea what the overall plan for our floor was. Focusing on my small part in making paper flowers tapped out my reserves of group enthusiasm. The morning of One Hundred Days there was a floor announcement. Everyone was to gather for hanging the decorations after lunch. I think Susan and I thought we would do this. She may have even joined them for some of it. I turned in my paper flowers and then got distracted somewhere else. The official showing was after dinner. Susan, Evelyn, and I ate together, and then went on a tour of the dorm floors.

Every six months there would be a graduating class reaching it's One Hundred Day marker. On that evening everyone took the ritual tour of the halls, everyone except those who were too laid back to participate. The women were never too sophisticated to assess other people's decorating skills. There was usually a spectacular floor that managed to outdo the others with an unparalleled surge of creativity. The competing floors always had to give in, and recognize the true superiority of the floor that had out-shone everyone. The countdown for One Hundred Days began with an artistic extravaganza. The drawback was that the show lingered on a long time, all one hundred days, at which time it would be disassembled in a party frenzy.

For three months we would live in a creative ensemble that resembled a senior prom gone awry. The tape would begin to dry out. Each piece, at its own rate, would lose its stickiness. Crepe paper streamers would stretch and sag, turning into nooses for all but the very short. Colors would fade. Clever anecdotes became grating. Finally, people would lose their reverence, and the defacing would begin. I was always relieved when it got to this stage. At least now the scenery would begin to take on some new and intriguing messages.

While the preparations were being made to decorate the halls, people were singularly preparing a private decoration. These were the posters I had noticed the first day of school. They were known as Goal Posters, but the name never made sense to me. What they were, was a large congratulation card to one's self. Students glued on pictures of their family and/or friends and wrote things like "YEAH WE DID IT!"

Some people made very personal statements thanking God or loved ones for their support. Evelyn and I talked about whether we were going to make Goal Posters. I thought they were the stupidest things in the world, and of course, would never be caught dead making one. Evelyn said she was considering it. This shocked me. Making personal statements in public was not usually an Evelyn-type activity. She felt she might have something to say, and was giving it some thought.

I began thinking about it too. If I were going to make one, what would I say regarding how I felt about leaving here? I decided AMF YOYO was how I felt. When I left County, I would be leaving the school AMF YOYO. I had heard the term on 6A, during my rotation. Dr. Susan Blade had a key chain with her unit keys on it. She carried the set of keys around constantly, her nervous fingers frequently toying with it. It was impossible to miss Mr. Grant's leather working skills, so I knew he had made it for her.

In block letters with scrolls on them, AMF YOYO was stamped into the leather. The letters were surrounded with flowers and painted bright colors. There was something incongruous about the combination of Hallmark colored flowers and those ominous looking letters. Every day I tried possible words to fit, I never got a match. No one would give me a direct answer to my question. I was in a staff meeting one morning and I finally heard Dr. Blade announce "We're sending this one home, AMF YOYO."

"Will somebody tell me what it means?" I must have finally demanded it with enough force because a resident explained, "It means, Adios Mother Fucker, You're On Your Own." It was an epithet for kids who for one reason or another had come as far as they were going to in this place, and needed to be cut loose. Sometimes it referred to a patient who wanted nothing to do with the unit, and had gone to court to get released. Other times it was for a teenager who had turned his/her life around, gained control, and was ready to re-enter the world. It meant the staff had done all that they could do; it was now up to the individual. For the kid who had been a pain in the ass it meant, "So long, you are no longer our problem." For the kid who had come a long way, it was more of a salute of confidence, his own should see him through.

The latter was how I felt about leaving County. County had done for me what she could; from here on I was on my own. I saw it as a badge of pride and courage. I was ready to accept the responsibility and challenge. The school was pulling back her protective arms, and pushing me out into the real world. AMF YOYO spoke to the fear that I had, that I would not do well, and to the courage I was needing to move forward with strength into this transition.

It was a mix of very solitary feelings I was having. Friends were there as supporters and comrades, but I had walked into County alone, and that was how I faced the wards each day. My experience here was nearing an end; what I had made of it was my personal choice. I was tremendously proud of myself. I had done things I never thought I could do. AMF YOYO spoke silently to me of the confidence I had to move forward.

I decided to make a Goal Poster. Usually they were large statements to the world, about three feet by four feet in size. My statement was very private; no one outside of 6A seemed to be familiar with the term. I found a five by seven inch picture of myself that Michael had taken on our camping trip. It seemed very appropriate. I am sitting on a boulder by the fire wearing three layers of coats and a wool hat. My hands are wrapped around a cup of hot chocolate for warmth and reassurance. My huge borrowed back pack is lying on the ground beside me, ready to be re-shouldered and moved along.

I glued the picture to an eight by ten piece of cardboard, and underneath in block letters I wrote, "N. BOAND, AMF YOYO." I taped my small poster onto a pillar at eye level, by the front of the lobby. I saw it several times every day, for one hundred days. My courage and confidence took a lift every time I looked at it. At the end of our one hundred days I went down and carefully removed my poster.

Graduation was now only three months away. I think that we instinctivly knew the two year friendships we had created in the midst of an enclosed world like County, stood very little chance of surviving in the outside. None of us would really talk about this. We were ticking off our days together on the calendar, and stubbornly refusing to acknowledge the emotional implications. The bonds between us were losing their glue as fast as the tape holding up our streamers.

Instead, as we moved toward our final eight week rotation, we talked about the future, where we would live, where we would work. Some people did make shared plans. After graduation, two or three new nurses planned to share an apartment, and work at the same hospital. My friends and I were not starting out as beginners in the work world. We were all independent. We had our own agendas for our lives. We could tell, as each of us described our plans, that we were headed for very divergent paths upon graduation. We talked about all of this as we rushed forward into the shortest eight weeks of our lives, but we never attempted to say good-bye.

Chapter Twenty-Eight

Into The Night

The time had arrived for our final rotation, Team Leading. Norman had split our group in half. Myself and three others were returning to Infected Orthopedics. This last rotation took place on the evening shift. We were to report on the wards at three p.m, and work until eleven p.m. I hated the idea of working past nine in the evening. Some things I can do after nine o'clock in the evening. I can eat, sit through a very engaging movie, or I can stay awake for the second half of a play, if it's good. But, I rarely attempt anything requiring intense concentration after nine p.m.

Once it becomes completely dark, and everyone under seven years old is asleep, my brain waves begin to diminish. At this point in the night I stop handling sharp objects and I attempt to avoid life-changing decisions. I was greatly concerned about handling IV's for thirty patients on antibiotics after ten p.m. The idea of pouring and distributing ten o'clock meds to the entire unit didn't thrill me either. I felt my chances of killing someone went up proportionately to the lateness of the evening.

There was no avoiding it - everyone's final rotation was on the evening shift. I entered into the night with trepidation, concern and a great deal of caffeine. The only things for me that make coffee drinkable are tons of sugar, french vanilla bean ice cream, and a dash of Bailey's. The Bailey's was out of the question before going to work, and our refrigerator wouldn't keep ice cream frozen. I made do with sugar and cream, swallowing the bitter stuff as fast as I could.

Getting dressed in the afternoon, I had to put on a second tag under my name tag. This was a homemade job, and it said either Team Leader, or Team Member. I wore it on my chest opposite from my cowboy pin. Since these tags were homemade they varied from person to person. Some scrawled the words on a three by five card in blue ball-point pen, others got creative with flowers and hearts. My tags bore large block letters shining in five shades of day-glo markers.

I always preferred pinning on my Leader tag to my Team Member tag. On my leader days, I would feel an air of authority, and I would swell with a determination to lead well. I took the role of leader very seriously. I planned out my approach, and how I would utilize my team members. I wanted to be intelligent, fair, concise, creative, thorough, efficient, sympathetic, and incredibly effective. I wanted others to be awed by my leadership skills, which was probably my main weakness in team leading.

I didn't get to lead right off; I had to be a team member a couple of times first. Though my impatience grew, I was fortunate because I was able to watch and learn from other people's successes and failures. I observed a wishy-washy, weak leader, the worst possible kind. I saw the chaos, confusion, and lack of coordination brought on by a refusal to bite the bullet and lead. I also did my time under a "Mien Fuhrer" dictator. I spent the week detesting the bitch, but noting that she got the job done.

Finally it was time to take my first shot at team leading. I arrived on the wards eager and ready. My sad looking uniform hung on my body like it had been weighted down with bricks. Two years of constant washing and drying with four softener sheets had turned the stiff scratchy fabric into a limp rag. I still wore my cowboy pin with his steely glint shining out from above my left breast. The extra velvet ribbons on my cap, and my good looking cowboy, didn't make up for how lousy I felt in this uniform. To lift my spirits, I had taken to wearing a mint green lace garter belt with stockings under my dull dress. Combined with my raciest bikini underwear, I felt a little more like myself as I walked through the halls of County.

Cheryl South was there to give the change of shift report. She went through describing each patient's condition. She then turned to me, the team leader, to make the evening's assignments. This was a very tricky political task. I had realized this watching my cohorts struggling. There was one R.N. working on the unit on the evening shift. They also had one Licensed Vocational Nurse (L.V.N.) and several attendants depending on the evening. Medications and IV's had to be handled by an R.N. or a senior student nurse. An L.V.N. has less training than an R.N.; therefore the jobs that require greater nursing judgment are restricted to the R.N.'s. This meant that the L.V.N. was frequently given the most difficult jobs on the unit, like the three or four worst dressing changes. Each dressing change could take an hour, which resulted in a very tough shift.

Student nurses loved being assigned meds or IV's. The work required focus and attention, but it was clean, and not physically demanding or gross. The R.N.'s wanted these jobs too, and L.V.N.'s felt shafted if they were given all the toughest jobs. I would attempt diplomacy in my assignments. The clean jobs of meds and IV's I would split, one for an R.N. and one for a student nurse.

I would then divide up the patients' rooms between the two remaining student nurses, the L.V.N. and the attendants. Sometimes I would assign a very skilled L.V.N. the most difficult dressing changes, and then make it up to her by assigning the rest of her patient care to the attendants and student nurses. As the Leader, my job was to supervise. I would take detailed notes on everything that needed to be done for each patient. I would give people their assignments and their directions. I would then spend the rest of the evening, notebook in hand, roaming the unit making sure everything got done.

The realities of life on the wards sunk in very slowly for me. Settling for less than a job well done was the most difficult lesson for me to learn. Cheryl South was the one that had to deal with my horrors at the realities of nursing. I came to her with tales of things that absolutely must be corrected for the safety of the patients. I was sure she would take immediate action. For two weeks, I was the stone in Cheryl South's shoe.

It began the first Monday I was a team leader. We had two nursing students from a local city college working on the unit that evening. I discovered other nursing schools trained at County in the evenings, while County students trained there during the days. Malcolm and Linda told me they were senior students, and had finished most of their schooling. They had trained in a small community hospital and they were a little nervous at the idea of working at County. County nurses are snobs. I am sure I was a bit smug and cocky showing Malcolm and Linda the ropes. I told them not to worry, it was just some dressing changes, they could handle it. This is the accepted code for introducing student nurses to new horrors.

I had given out everyone's assignments. I checked my lists twice to make sure everything was covered, and began making my first pass through the unit to see where I was needed, and how everything was going. I entered the long room at the end of the hall where I had assigned Malcolm three patients with dressing changes. I had given him three very easy patients because the vacant look in his eyes had made me uneasy. Malcolm had studied the care plan for his first patient.

He had collected several sterile bundles that contained enough equipment to perform major surgery. He had rolled in a special table to the center of the room, eight feet away from his patient, to provide him a place to set up his sterile field. He had full bottles of alcohol, hydrogen peroxide, and normal saline, all with their caps on, sitting on the table. His equipment was still wrapped up in sterile bundles. Behind the table stood Malcolm. He had his hands straight up in the air wearing his sterile gloves, trying to keep them safe, while his face wore a look of absolute panic.

Malcolm saw me and announced, "I'm ready to go, I have everything, I've got my gloves on." I was speechless. I didn't know whether to be outraged at the incompetence, or to wet my pants with laughter. I think I was much closer to the latter, so I stayed silent, and focused on sphincter control. Malcolm became uneasy, waiting for me to speak. He squinted his eyes, and tried to read my face. He couldn't make out the expression I was wearing. I think he was trying to decide if I was dazzled by his flashy display, or terrified by his incompetence. I asked Malcolm, with as little sarcasm as possible, "How are you going to open all this stuff without contaminating your sterile gloves?" Malcolm didn't know what to do next.

I proceeded to introduce Malcolm to Mother Merlin's wonderful world of sterile technique. I performed the magic of turning green bundles into a sterile field ready for a dressing change. Then we each donned fresh sterile gloves and proceeded with the dressing changes he had been assigned. Watching Malcolm's face as we worked did not give me a great deal of hope for rapid improvement. I could tell by the look in his eyes the information just wasn't getting through. I did the first dressing change. He assisted me with the second. I suggested he do the third one. I would observe and help if needed. Help was needed, immediately, and throughout the third dressing change. I realized this wasn't Malcolm's fault. Somebody had assigned him to this unit without assessing his skills.

Once again I took my concerns for patient safety to the head nurse, Cheryl. I told her how shocking it was. This man had no skills; he was a danger on the unit. Cheryl already knew he was not very skilled. This was not the most shocking thing she had ever seen. Her plan of action was to keep Malcolm as far away from me as possible. She said she thought I worked better with other members of the team. She gave him menial work that wasn't too taxing. She would have someone watch out for Malcolm and see that he was getting along all right.

I don't know exactly what I expected Cheryl to do. Malcolm was a student nurse, not there to be hired or fired. Her only power over Malcolm was to tell him what to do; evaluating his progress was up to his instructor. I think I wanted her to be a heroine, to step forward, and purge this incompetent person from our profession. Cheryl wasn't looking for heroics. She was trying to run a difficult unit, and did an excellent job of it; she was a woman who understood prioritizing.

What slowly sunk in to my brain regarding nursing was that there is more to the job than giving excellent patient care. Getting along is important when working in a group situation. I discovered that no matter how well I did, and how much my supervisor might value me, she wouldn't go to bat for me against a group of employees that felt I didn't fit in. Causing turmoil in the ranks by requiring fellow employees to do better work does not create a happy team. One stellar employee can not replace a dozen disgruntled ones.

I learned some important things about myself in nursing, and a few of the seeds of understanding were sown in Team Leading. I learned I do my best work one-on-one. I take direction beautifully. I am an extremely conscientious supervisor and leader. I am only fun to work with for another serious worker. I learned that when the status quo is what works, I am probably not a very good person for the job. I learned that others don't necessarily value me for what I value in myself. And, in the long run, I am probably not a team player.

Chapter Twenty Nine

The Finishing Touches

    To begin with, we needed a song. Every graduating class had the job of picking out the music they wanted to use as their processional. The class before ours had real creative balls. They had chosen to march in to the theme from Star Wars. It set a jubilant tone for the day. This was a hard act to follow. I thought we really needed to stretch ourselves here. Bob Dylan's <u>Forever Young</u>, the <u>1812 Overture</u>, Springsteen's <u>Born to Run</u>, or the theme from "Bonanza" all seemed like pretty good options to me.
    On a Monday morning at eight a.m., just before lecture began, our class president stood up to make an announcement. Today we would hear and vote on samples of music to be used as our processional. She reminded us that this was a solemn, dignified event, and that the music should set an appropriate tone. My hope faded; this meant there was already a conspiracy underfoot to promote dull and pompous. A perfectly groomed young woman made a grand display of putting her tape into the machine. Our president nodded approvingly as she pushed the play button. It must have been a mistake, because out poured the saddest dirge of a song that I had ever heard.
    "What the hell is that?", I asked Evelyn. She is very informed about music, so to keep up her image, she told me it was classical. "Yes, I know that. Why would anyone want to march to it? We'll have to crawl down the aisle." This got our row going. We decided it was a funeral march to depict our grief at leaving County.
    Our president clarified for us that this beautiful and moving piece was the theme song from the movie, "Ordinary People." That explains it. This was a currently popular movie, very well done, about the death of one brother, and the suicidal effect it had on the remaining brother. Seemed like a perfect choice for a celebration of accomplishment and personal liberation. Our president spoke with dignity and authority in her voice. It was perfectly obvious where her feelings lay. As a side thought, Madame President asked if there were any other selections to be heard? God, I hoped so. My friends and I began to panic, somebody else must have come up with some music. A voice from the audience yelled out a complaint, "nobody told us we were supposed to bring music today."
    An unflappable Madame President maintained her dignified cool as she informed us, "This was announced several weeks ago. Today is the only day available for this. You should have read the bulletin board." Several obscene suggestions regarding the bulletin board and her person flew back at her, which she chose to ignore. We were doomed; she had us. A couple of other people played songs, both better than the first, and we enthusiastically supported these.

Complaints were registered about the somber tone of the first piece and the desire for something more upbeat. But it was all a formality. The class voted as their leader had suggested. We in the back two rows made the suggestion that the class get knee pads to avoid rug burns as we crawled down the aisle. As usual, we were ignored.

This conflict between factions began way back in the initial semester of school. The first act of solidarity for every entering class was to design a class pin. This was not the fourteen karat gold school pin we would receive on graduation. This was a pin unique to each class in gold colored metal. It was worn throughout the two years of nursing school. I had thought Leonardo da Vinci's anatomical man was a good symbol for us. The pin would measure about an inch and a half by one inch in size. I thought the nude male figure symbolizing man in a state of health and balance was a nice touch for nursing.

Voting was to take place around the end of the first month at County. Four designs had been submitted to the class. Two of the designs were total confused nonsense, and no real challenge to da Vinci. The other suggestion was a replica of Florence Nightingale's lamp, the standard symbol of nursing. Well, all hell broke lose when some of the girls realized that I was suggesting putting a likeness of male genitals on their pins. Actually they were trend setters, way ahead of their time. They beat the current trend of censorship in art by almost ten years. There was an uproar, and people immediately took sides. The progressive thinkers were determined, the lamp had been overdone to death. Besides, on a pin whose entire length measures an inch and a half, the issue of genitals being depicted was ridiculous.

It became an issue of balls, would we have them or not. The vote was close, but the answer was no. We ended up with the lamp. The loss of the anatomical man was hard to take, but women and elephants never forget. Not more than a week after we had learned that we would be slogging down the aisles to a deathly tune, our graduating class annual made its debut. The young women who put the annual together were of a more creative bent. They also had a sense of humor and closure. The cover was white and bore a reproduction of da Vinci's anatomical man in black. The genitals alone were almost an inch in length. Finally, we had gotten some balls.

A couple of events had to take place before graduation. One of these was our emergency drill. This was an event for the entire class of one hundred. It was designed to expand and test our skill in handling emergency situations. I don't understand exactly where they thought we had picked up this knowledge of handling emergencies. We had all taken seventy-two hours of CPR training, and had been certified. But a single heart attack or a choking kid is a long way from a hoard of injured, panicked, and dying people.

We had no real emergency training, no class with that title. Somehow, it was assumed that we had absorbed through our pores a secret known only to those in the healing arts, how to handle a mad, chaotic and injured crowd. They did show us a film, Disaster in a Hospital, or some such title. The film was set in a hospital much like County. Something went awry, and a fire was started.

Kaboom, the whole hospital was going up in flames. This film was almost as gruesome as the ones on giving birth. Nurses ran through the hospital doing what needed to be done to move the immobile patients. Traction lines were cut with scissors, legs came crashing down while patients screamed in pain. Patients were heaved to the floor on sheets, then dragged down the halls. The nurse with the medication keys grabbed the pain meds and headed out the door.

This was a shocking, disturbing film. The thought of a hospital fire was horrifying. But I was glad I saw it. If ever I was caught in that situation my mind now understood what must be done. You cut the lines, bang a head on the floor, just get them out. You deal with the ramifications afterwards. That's why the nurse had taken the pain meds. The problem was they weren't going to run us through a fire emergency. Our emergency was going to be a surprise. We drew lots for the roles we were to be assigned.

I unfolded my small square of paper to see the word "Victim," a time, nine a.m., and a location, somewhere in the hills above Pasadena. I was so glad I hadn't gotten "Doctor" or "Triage Nurse," because these people had to know what they were doing. Victim was great. I could just lie around, role-playing pain and agony. Secretly, I have always wanted to act; I think I could do it. I can moan, groan and convulse, go into shock or hysterics, simultaneously if you like. The neat thing about being a victim is that it's impossible to screw up, especially if you understand the signs and symptoms of your injury. If in doubt, shock is always a perfect standby.

I was prepared for my role because I had done this before. Michael was a Red Cross volunteer training emergency medical technicians. I was a volunteer victim for one of their graduation drills. I shocked out beautifully, even controlling my breathing, to the point of freaking out a pre-graduate EMT. When he threatened to give me mouth to mouth, I stopped role playing, and told him to back off.

I gave myself thirty minutes for the drive from County to the drill site. It was a Saturday morning, so I figured there wouldn't be any traffic. I never really give myself enough time to get anywhere. I may correctly estimate driving time, but I never include the five minutes it takes to find my keys and purse. I think people who are always late are late because they don't like to be early. I didn't disappoint myself that day; I was at least fifteen to twenty minutes late. I consider fifteen minutes to be pretty much on time, so I wasn't doing too badly. This was a very strange place. The sheriffs used it for one of their training centers during the week. The area was made up of barren rolling hills, standard arid California landscape. There were partial buildings (made up of foundations, with two or three sides, framed doorways and windows without glass) scattered around the three to four acres that we were going to use. Several of the buildings already had fresh, hand-painted signs on them saying "Hospital," "School," "Morgue," etc.

I was greeted abruptly by an instructor, "You're late, you're a victim right? He's doing the make-up over there." That's the other good thing about being a victim, you get to wear neat make-up. Michael had done a wonderful job making me look dreadful for the Red Cross drill. It would have made sense, if I had given it any thought, that Michael would be making up the victims today. I walked in the direction indicated until I turned a corner, and came upon Michael, surrounded by his make-up equipment and eager victims. I waited my turn in line while my stomach tensed, uncertain of his reaction. Michael was a professional volunteer, and he treated me appropriately. He was friendly, pleasant and tried to make me feel more comfortable. I would never again be completely comfortable around Michael; the pain between us had been too intense. Nor would the affection between us wane completely.

Through the magic of latex, glue, and make-up, Michael created a gory looking open wound with a piece of bone jutting out of my upper thigh. My leg looked totally gross, dripping with blood, exposed bone, and heavy bruises. Michael finished his job by giving me a fully shocked face. A thin shadow of blue-gray grease paint hung around my eyes, mouth, and cheeks. My face was then lightly sponged with glycerin to create beads of sweat.

I was the last victim finished. The supervisors of the drill hustled me over to one of the partial buildings. On my way to the building, I saw a sign that had been posted near the parking lot. The sign announced, "An earthquake took place at nine forty-five this morning." The rest of the students were due to arrive at ten o'clock, five minutes from now. I assumed this was all the information they were going to receive.

The building I was located in had three walls, no roof, and framed doors and windows. The observers of the drill kept track of how many victims were located in each spot. This way they could rate the efficiency of the others in finding us, and hopefully not leave any victims lying around undiscovered and left behind when the drill was over.

I didn't want to be left baking in the sun any longer than necessary. As soon as possible, I wanted to be resting in the lap of luxury with sweet nurses surrounding me, taking care of my every need. I wanted to be comfortably injured. I stepped over a couple of other victims sprawled out on the dirt floor. As one of the observers yelled out, "Places everyone", I climbed up on a window sill and leaned back on it making myself as comfortable as possible. I also made sure to have my gory leg beautifully exposed. Nothing gets the attention of people in an emergency drill like a good gooey wound. I was thankful I had brought a book to read while I sat there waiting to be discovered.

While my fellow victims were lying on the ground in the sun, I sat in the window frame reading. I was smarter than I had realized. Our rescuers' rush to our sides took over half an hour. Eventually our classmates showed up and began wandering around the site. They were wearing ID badges, and expressions of confused curiosity. When the first rescuer appeared in the framed doorway of our building, on cue, we victims let loose with a cacophony of moans, groans, and wails of pain. Howling with pain is not my style. I indulged in low groans and gasps. Rescuers tend to go for the noisiest and the bloodiest. There was too much noise to compete with, I let my gory leg and shocky face do my bidding.

Screamers get on everybody's nerves, and there is always someone who feels compelled to play this role. I guess its a good thing, since real life disasters tend to produce an hysteric or two. Surprisingly, I don't remember anyone that day by name other than Michael. It was something about the effect of the drill. We were ourselves until the moment it happened. As soon as that first rescuer appeared in our doorway, we became victims, totally absorbed with our part in this play. The students discovering our mangled bodies and minds were confused only briefly. We watched them spontaneously transform into the role their ID tag announced. Throughout the exercise I never saw anyone break character. It was surprising considering we had all known each other for two years; the site was littered with best friends and buddies.

The emergency team entering our door consisted of a man and two women. He was clearly in a leader role. He pointed to the screamer and yelled, "Get her out of here." We were all relieved to see the mad woman removed. Now my soft moans and shallow breathing could be heard and appreciated. Immediately the remaining female rescuer rushed to my side. She promptly began soothing my anxiety, and buying herself time to think. "It's OK, you're going to be alright."

She was good, I was impressed. The site of my leg took her back, but she held together and did all the right stuff. She recognized the signs of shock and the need for immediate intervention. From here on out the drill was a breeze for me. A paper pretend IV was started in my arm, and I was gently helped to the hospital. A limited number of paper cards with the word stretcher on them were handed out to rescuers. Stretcher was now pinned to my chest as two attendants walked me to the area labeled hospital. Here I got more of a sense of how the drill was run. Everything was available in limited supply. Three by five cards were marked saline IV, blood, penicillin, bandage, whatever might be needed. Students had to figure out how to use their resources.

In the hospital I was given a cot to lie down on while my doctors and nurses debated whether I needed blood, antibiotics, or surgery. I needed all three, so the game continued. They typed my blood, and loaded me up on penicillin. In real life, I am allergic to penicillin, so I figured now was a good time to show them my version of anaphylactic shock. I gasped, choked and stopped breathing. I began to convulse. They got it. "She's having an allergic reaction to the penicillin, get some epinephrine." My classmates were really very good; we must know more than I thought we knew.

I watched everything intently, absorbed with our drama. I observed everyone's actions to see if I would have overlooked something they caught, or what would I choose to do differently. I spent the rest of the afternoon watching the drill from the vantage point of a hospital cot. It was a great place for an overall view of the action. By the end of the day I had learned quite a bit from the students who had spent their evenings working on the County emergency wards. You could pick out the ones who had chosen this area as their specialty. It was their time to shine and share with us all they had learned. I watched and absorbed, trying to memorize everything I could. If there was a disaster out there looming in my future, I wanted to be as efficient and prepared as possible. In reality, if I was in a disaster, I would probably end up over in the corner assigned the job of containing the crazy screamers.

Following the emergency drill there were two more County traditions that had to take place before we would walk down that aisle to our terrible music and receive our diplomas. First, The County Board of Supervisors wanted to fete us. This was done for every graduating class. A lovely luncheon for all the members of our class would be held at the Los Angeles Music Center, which was pretty fancy for a bunch of students living in forty dollar a month rooms and existing on County food. They were even providing us with transportation. Several County busses would be available to take us to and from the luncheon. These were the same Pepto Bismal pink busses that the Sheriffs used to haul prisoners, barred windows and everything.

Almost everyone I knew felt going to a free luncheon was a good idea. A few of the men thought a tie was too much effort, so they passed. But most of the women didn't mind a chance to put on nice clothes and be fed free food, even if we did have to buy our own wine. There was some discussion as to how we wanted to arrive. Driving one's own car had infinitely more class than arriving in a pink, fully-barred bus. Susan, Evelyn, Sam and I went back and forth on this issue. Evelyn and Susan favored the bus. It would be easy, free, and one could start partying even before take off. Sam is a man with style; he was thinking valet parking. I was leaning toward Sam's direction until we realized none of us had any idea where in the Center this deal was to be held.

I ended up signing the ride sheet for the bus with the rest of my friends. The afternoon of the luncheon Susan and I opened our doors so we could talk while we dressed. I got into the frig and pulled out a bottle of wine. Silk dresses, high heels, and a County prisoner bus require wine to be compatible. I found my opener and began to pry out the cork. I called out to Susan, "I'm pouring us some wine, why don't you call Evelyn?" That was how we began our farewell congratulatory luncheon at County, trying on various shoe and stocking combinations, doing and re-doing our hair, and drinking wine.

We were The Graduating Seniors. We could do as we damn well pleased. Toasting ourselves, and slightly toasted, the colorful array of flowers that made up the women of our class descended the elevators and stairs to gather in the lobby, creating one wild bouquet. The men that were present were overpowered. Their navy, gray, and brown suits disappeared in a sea of early summer dresses. Men in suits usually feel like they must behave. Women in light summer dresses feel the sun on their skin, and the breeze on their legs and are enlivened. We three were not the only ones to have begun our celebration while putting on our make-up. The lobby filled with women who bubbled, and sparkled, and smelled divine.

All this loveliness was split up into groups, formed into lines, and marched out to the waiting busses. Someone had been kind enough to clean the busses out, so the smell wasn't too bad. Within moments of getting on, people were wiggling their fingers out through the bars and open windows, waving at everyone they could. We were monkeys in a cage, and behaved with about equal decorum. Sam had opted out of the bus experience. It was just too far beneath his dignity. After all of the discussion, I just couldn't pass up the chance to ride around in a silk dress, on a prisoner bus, on my way to a ladies' luncheon.

The windows were locked in a three inch down position. Our hair was blown to bits by the time we got off of the freeway. The luncheon was standard banquet fare - chicken and rice with sauce and green peas. Most of us purchased another glass of wine. The speeches were boring, and by people we had never seen before who made decisions about how our tax dollars were spent. It seemed pretty obvious to me, the dollars were spent giving lunches for graduating nursing students. Not a bad return on their money, considering all the hours of free labor we had given to County.

I hadn't really considered this aspect of our time spent at County; that we had provided free labor. I had never thought of any of the work I had done there as a service. I considered it a learning experience that I had paid for. I had spent all those hours on the units working to get it right, wanting to do it perfectly. Perfection is an impossible goal in the best of circumstances; in a county hospital it becomes quixotic. It wasn't until graduation time that I became aware of this concept of seeing ourselves as free labor. Our yearbook is even dedicated to this notion. Our editor dedicated it to ourselves, the graduating seniors, and "the countless hours of service" we had given to County.

Seeing my work there as a service I gave for free gives it a noble ring. However, this is a concept that I can not really embrace. I didn't do it as a service, or a gift. I did it to learn things I wanted to know. If it was a gift to anyone, it was a costly, difficult one, given to myself. The pride I felt in my accomplishment was absolutely tremendous. I had no trouble joining in with the rest of the class and the Board of Supervisors in saluting our achievement. A luncheon seemed absolutely appropriate to me. If they wanted to, they could give a parade.

The last event before our graduation day was an unofficial ceremony that always took place the final night on the wards. Most of us had never been to a prior class' graduation ceremony, but we dorm dwellers had lived through the last night on the wards with three previous classes. We knew what was expected of us, a night of acting out and total debauchery. We planned to do our best.

It had finally come, our last night of working on the County units as student nurses. For some, this was merely the transition to the role of a paid R.N. For others, myself included, it was truly the end of a unique period in our lives. I had no intention of ever returning to medical nursing after this night. I was moving on to the psychiatric hospital, Unit 6A, across the street. Across the street was the same as around the world, the two were so different. I had done my time in medical nursing. I had suctioned, intubated, emptied bed pans, and changed massive dressings. None of my sensory organs had escaped untouched. I had not injured, maimed, or killed anyone. I did not stop to contemplate, to savor this last moment with the pseudomonias infections and the penicillin bottles. I was ready to party with my pals and get the hell out of there.

We were all still on the evening shift, working from three to eleven p.m. Getting dressed for this last evening took a little extra care. This was because of another tradition. The rule was, when the graduating seniors returned to the dorm after finishing their last shift, other students would grab them, and rip their uniforms off their backs. It was sort of an opening call to the festivities; forcibly stripping the seniors. They weren't gentle about it either; nobody bothered with buttons - we're talking rrrrrip.

The question that occurred to me as I dressed was, what did I want to be left standing in once my uniform was torn to shreds? Then again my dress might remain intact. It was the social types who were totally shredded. Not hanging out with the younger girls, and seeming somewhat aloof, it was possible that no one would lay a hand on me. I was sure they wouldn't dare touch Evelyn, and maybe not even Susan. So I might not get shredded at all. How would I feel about that?

A sane, rational person would feel good about that. It's pretty tough to rip someone's uniform off their back with out injuring their body to some small degree. It would be much more dignified to slip into my room and change into some jeans, putting an end to the whole question. This was certainly an option chosen by some. I wanted the whole experience though. I wanted my uniform obnoxiously torn from my body just like it had been from hundreds of nursing students before me. It was a romantic attachment to all those who had preceded me, and to those who would follow. It seemed like a part of the pageant.

I wasn't sure how to guarantee that I would be part of the pageant. It's supposed to be spontaneous. You are supposed to try to avoid it. Ah, but you can't, you are grabbed and the girls do the ugly deed, ignoring your protests. I decided the heck with spontaneity, if there was a chance of my uniform being ripped off, I wanted to look attractive underneath. I decided on my mint green lace garter belt and matching bikinis. I had given up wearing bras on the unit my second month of school; they made me cranky. Instead I wore a full slip with lace embroidered cups, a small pink bow, and rose buds; pretty busy, but sweet. Garter belts look hot with spiky high heels; with clunky white nursing shoes the effect was shifted to the weird. I slipped into my shabbiest uniform, and pinned my student cap to my head for the last time.

The nursing staff was prepared for us that night. They had seen enough of these "last evenings" to expect little work from us. We were assigned light case loads that required little mental rigor. Things seemed pretty normal until about nine o'clock then the visits began. I was beginning to get disappointed thinking this was going to be just like any other night on the units. I was hoping for something special, something memorable. That's when I heard the loud clanging of stairwell doors, followed by shrieks of laughter. A gang of senior girls was rampaging the units, and attacking everyone with tape.

Each nursing station kept a variety of colored tape on hand. The tape was used for color coding different types of stuff. The nursing students were now busy color coding everyone they could get their hands on. Some had spelled out messages on their backs in bright tape. I hung around the periphery, smiling at their wild behavior, and worrying that they might be yelled at for wasting County tape supplies. One of the younger women grabbed me, and yelled, "here Nicole, let me do your back." Some others gathered around, and helped her.

Popcorn appeared, along with Cokes, and some illicit champagne. While several worked on my back, others were madly applying tape to any object coming within their range. Finally, I was spun around, and pushed toward a mirror. Cranking my head back over my shoulder, I could read it in reverse. My back bore bright green letters six inches high, AMF YOYO. I loved it. It was the only reference anyone had made to my goal poster; it couldn't have pleased me more.

The next hour or so on the unit was a blur. We were marking time until eleven o'clock. The clock finally pushed its hands up in surrender, and we were free. That's it, no more, all done, we're out of here! An unruly gang of marauding senior nurses made their way back to the dorm. No sleep tonight. Senior nurses always have their last day on wards during the middle of the week. It is a curse that is perpetrated upon underclassmen, preferably on days when they have a test the next morning. The earliest arrivals could already be seen dashing in their underwear back to their rooms, or roaming the halls in their slips, beer in one hand, shredded uniform in the other.

Still things were under control, it wasn't too wild yet. I got off the elevator on my floor, and saw two seniors being jumped in the central lounge area. It seemed kind of pathetic for me to stand around waiting to be jumped. I figured it wasn't going to happen, and I headed down the hall to my room. I heard the cry, "There's Nicole, get her." I didn't even have time to think, "oh boy". Hands grabbed me, and began ripping at my uniform. My sleeve was torn right off. Buttons scattered over the floor. Some female gorilla managed to grab a hold of the back of my dress, and tear the whole section clean away. Every bit of disgust we had for these uniforms was poured out on the dresses being torn from the backs of the seniors.

Looking back at the scene in my mind, I see no men present. Historically this was a ritual that took place among all women. The men had broken ground, and had moved in to join us in our territory, but I don't think they felt quite comfortable in the forcible removal of clothes from the women students. It was a good move on their part. There are some events and traditions that just can't make a graceful shift to co-ed. Men also don't seem comfortable ripping clothing off one another. Too bad, it was fun.

What the men did do was get down and party on the fourth floor. Serious, heavy party! Quatro Flats was fired up and going strong by the time I put on some jeans and got down there. Our class was known to have some rowdy folks. The required attitude on exiting the elevator doors was "what the fuck." This was the end of the seventies, the beginning of the eighties. The administration had not yet declared its war on drugs. Nancy Reagan was years away from coming up with her slogan, "Just say no." This was a crowd with a liberal sprinkling of what is euphemistically called recreational users, and tonight they were going to recreate.

The elevator doors opened onto a dark, smoke-filled hall with heavy metal music blaring. The hallway went in two directions, but everything that was happening was happening down on the left, where all of the men in our class lived. Those who were pleased to have the party pour into their rooms left their doors open. Over half of the doors were open, with crowds of people moving in and out of the doorways. I knew where to find my friends, down at Gregory's place, a major hot spot. I made my way to Gregory's room where the celebration was in full swing.

"Nicole, I have something for you to drink!" This was a sweet welcome from Gregory, because all any of these people ever drink is beer. I can't stand the taste of beer, so I would always be the one at a gathering who sat without a drink, or sipping water. Eventually I would get hungry, or thirsty, and head upstairs to my room for some Nestle's Quik. Tonight Gregory was grinning, and waving champagne at me. "I know you won't say no to this." I stepped over and around the crowd, and made my way into his arms. There was a big kiss, a squeeze, and a tall glass of sparkling, bubbly, cheap stuff.

A crowd of about twenty to thirty people packed Gregory's tiny room. A primitive, chanting dance was going on in the center. There was an absence of free chairs, so for a while I plopped in Susan's lap. The words we spoke have been blurred away by the music, the bodies, the pounding, and the smell of pot wafting through the air above us. An insistent yelling brought the room to attention. Michael had climbed up onto a chair, and was trying to make an announcement. Finally the group caught on, and politely contained itself. The party, the noise, the dance, were all held in abatement for the moment.

Michael stood solemn and erect, a bottle of expensive whisky in his hand. "My dear friend and mentor John Goodin gave me this bottle when I was accepted into nursing school. He told me to have a drink on him when I graduated. Tonight, I would like you to join me in a toast to my friend John." A normal person would not have tried to orchestrate a serious moment with a group like this, but Michael was not a normal person; he was extraordinary and dramatic. His sincerity was not to be mocked. It took people a moment to shift, and to realize sincere emotion was being requested of them, not an easy thing to call forth from a group blindly doing the bump in the dark, and howling to the music.

A generosity of heart prevailed. Someone in the crowd yelled, "To John!" This was something one could dance to if given a beat. The beat was supplied by the constant echoes of the call, "To John!" The celebratory chant took hold, bodies swayed and feet stomped to the rhythm. Michael stood on the chair, sipping a glass of the whisky, his private moment exalted. Meanwhile, the bottle made the rounds of the room, each person taking a swig and shouting, "To John!" The bottle finally reached me. I swallowed and yelled, "To John, and to Michael!" The roar of the crowd obscured my toast completely.

I was beginning to get claustrophobic, so I decided to prowl around, and see what was happening in some of the other rooms. I walked into the hallway, and encountered two of our prissiest instructors. These were both nice ladies, but very straight and prim. A third instructor exited a room across the hall whispering excitedly, "You won't believe what's in there. He's got an eight inch pile of hash just sitting on the sink. Its like a buffet." I was surprised that the women weren't appalled. They were just like me, curious. I wanted to see what an eight inch pile of hash looked like, and so did they.

Of course I wasn't included in this conversation; I was eavesdropping. Now I planned to nonchalantly tail them into the room and see if I could spot the hash. The door was open, and there were about ten people in the room milling around. The required music was blaring away. No one was standing near the sink. I watched these two nursing instructors timidly attempt a casual stroll by. One was determined; she was going to see what this stuff looked like. They made their quick pass by, practically holding hands for moral support. They barely cleared the door before they broke into excited giggles, "Did you see it? Did you see it?"

Well I hadn't seen it yet, and I wanted to. There was no possible excuse I could use to cruise the sink area other than to take a look, or to take a hit. The heck with it, I'll just walk over, and take a look. The mystique of it was amazing. It was as if the nurses and I were taking a peek inside a window to watch a live sex show. I was hoping someone would walk over, and use some, so I could watch. I wondered what the etiquette was around helping yourself to someone's hash. Was this a buffet? Or was this more of a personal display of wealth, like setting out your Baccarat crystal for guests to admire? No one in the room showed any interest in the hash, so my questions remained unanswered. All there was left to do was to take a look. And it was no big deal, just a perfect little mound of what looked like dark brown dirt. If you didn't know it was worth a lot of money, you would assume it was something for the dust buster to take care of.

It was nearing two in the morning, and the celebrators were getting ready to move on to phase two, the orgy. The orgy is much more of a phantom than a reality. It went on the principle that if you were really cutting loose, and being truly wild, you would probably have sex with someone that you normally wouldn't let touch you, or perhaps someone you had secretly desired for ages. In reality, most people were so tired by that time that they wanted to go to bed alone, or with the one they loved.

When the call to orgy came it was greeted by most with looks of "don't be ridiculous." I have noticed it's never the most appealing people who want to orgy, it's the ones you really don't care to see in their birthday suits. I might even feel differently about it if Robert Redford, Cary Grant, and Kevin Costner walked into my living room and cried "Let's orgy." I doubt it, but at least I might take a few more minutes to consider it.

In the following days the gossip came around of the straggling few who had attempted the ritual orgy. It was a sign that the times were changing. The sixties and early seventies would never return. The atmosphere just wasn't right for an orgy any more. The joy of it was gone, and all that was left was the work. I was told they finally just gave up, and fell asleep on the floor.

As it was, at two a.m. I headed for bed, alone. Jeff wasn't around. Tonight had been a night to celebrate with my peers, my comrades in bed pans and bedsores. I walked off the medical wards that night with no desire to ever return, and the feeling remains. Most went to sleep that night content in the thought that when they returned to the units it would be as a staff nurse. I went to sleep thanking the universe for the psychiatric unit 6A.

Chapter Thirty

Pomp and Circumstance

The day to let our families, friends, and loved ones salute our accomplishments had finally arrived. This day we would make the final transition out of the role of student nurses and become graduate nurses. We would have to wait until we passed our state board exams before California would grant us the title of licensed R.N., but until then, graduate nurse looked very good. I had been through two graduation ceremonies previously, for high school and college. I had taken both events for granted as your standard ceremonial stuff. I had assumed all along that I would graduate from high school and college, so neither seemed very special or unique to me. However, as I stood in the shower washing my hair in preparation for the celebration, I felt a slow building sense of something new to me. I finished blow drying my hair, and putting on my make-up, as the feeling intensified. By the time I got to my mascara, I could identify it. Pride!

I had felt pride before. I felt it about a couple of art pieces I had done in high school. I felt it after flawlessly clearing a round of jumps on horseback. I even felt pride over not having voted for Nixon. But these were small swellings of pride. What was happening here today was big, bold, screaming pride. I couldn't believe it. I didn't even feel shy about feeling this stuffed full of myself. I leaned into the mirror in Jeff's bathroom putting on my lipstick, and was nearly blinded by the intense light beaming from my face. I was aglow, an incredibly beautiful way to look. Whoever decided pride was a sin was surely out to discourage the best in mankind. Who would not want this feeling? Who would not want it for their child?

The glow didn't even dim as I put on my freshly polished orthopedic nursing shoes and my funky nursing uniform. Sam was due to pick me up in a few minutes. For the last time I carefully made the dopey little pin curl on the top of my head that we all used to anchor our caps. This time it was a fresh, pristine cap, a graduate nurses' cap, with a black velvet stripe running all the way around the brim. I petted my cap and caressed it. I studied it from every angle in the mirror. This was the only time I would ever wear it. To me, it looked supremely stunning.

I opened a tiny two inch square jewelry box, and gently removed my gold pin. This was my GRADUATION PIN. We had heard about it for two years, dreamed of it, yearned for it, and now I held it in my hand. I held it gently because Evelyn's broke the first time she played with her's. I didn't want the same sad experience. I turned it over, and admired my initials and graduation date carved in the back. That was part of the bummer if it broke. They had replaced Evelyn's pin with a new one, but they wouldn't fork out for having the new one engraved. She got stuck with a generic County pin. I attached the pin to my uniform in the approved place, above my left breast. My final grooming act was to pin my tin cowboy onto my collar. He had sat through all the stench, and the muck, and the guck with me; now it was time to march down the aisle and get our diploma. I kissed Jeff good bye, reminded him where to meet me after the ceremony and headed out to the curb.

Almost immediately Sam pulled up in his green bug. Waiting for me on the seat was a small package. "A graduation, and an I'm going to miss you gift." The truth finally comes out. I begin crying telling him I will miss him too. So much for the mascara; I should have known better. Sam handed me a hanky. I opened the box to find a pair of small salt and pepper shakers each in the shape of a cockatiel. It took me a minute to realize they were in honor of Chromina, my hide and seek bird. The tears started again, and I kept on soaking Sam's handkerchief.

It seemed to me the organizers were getting us here awfully early, almost two hours before the guests. I couldn't imagine what would take them that long to set up. It ended up nothing took them that long, they hadn't trusted we could get ourselves to the place on time, so they got us here an hour early. We found Evelyn, Susan, Gregory, and Sharon roaming around the auditorium steps, complaining of the early hour. There was a subdued, muted feeling, as singularly we all contemplated the significance of the day, and the upcoming changes in our lives.

It was too difficult to stand at the auditorium and wait. The six of us decided to cross the street to a hotel and have some coffee. We forcibly murdered the next hour and a half with tea and coffee, just to make it go away. By the time we made it back to the auditorium, we had to rush to find our places and prepare ourselves for the entrance processional. Before we began, I quickly looked for Michael. I found him standing alone. I congratulated him on his graduation, and he returned the sentiment to me. The barriers were down for a moment. It was our good-bye. Both of us wished the other well. I believe it was mutually heartfelt. It was warm and respectful.

Our senior instructors were the ones who arranged us for the ceremony. They had made an effort to note who was friends with whom. The seating was arranged accordingly. Gilbert Richardson made sure Sam and I would be seated to together. My marching partner would be Susan. Suite mates to marching mates, it seemed perfectly fitting. As our sad, slow song began to pour forth from the amplifiers, we jostled for position and started our stately march down the aisle.

The entire auditorium was packed with the families and friends of the graduates. I looked around, stretching to my full height, wondering if I would be able to spot my family. I don't know what I was thinking. My family is the least innocuous gang of personalities ever to assemble. While I craned my neck around searching the far reaches of the room, under my nose the yelling began, "Nicole, Nicole, Nicole!" They have never let me down at a ceremony. When their presence is requested, they always show up in full verbal force. I blushed, waved, made eye contact with each one of them. Flash bulbs began blinding me. Jeff was taking my picture. My oldest sister and my father were taking my picture. My other sister got off a shot of me. I began to feel immensely silly in this dopey outfit. I was also being pushed from behind. I waved to my own personal crowd of groupies, and headed up the stairs to my seat on stage.

Here Susan and I parted, and Sam replaced her sitting next to me. The speeches began. I feel I should pay my family for all the times they have had to sit through ceremonial speeches, to demonstrate their love, and support for me. I have recently promised them, no more degrees. However, some of the speeches were good. Especially the ones by the students. They spoke of pride in one's self, in our classmates, and in our profession. I was so full of pride that day, I had plenty to spare for everyone.

I listened to the part of the speeches I liked - the descriptions of how hard we had worked, of all we had learned, how far we had come, and especially, how much we had changed. The speakers finally gave way, and a chorus line of graduates presented us with a musical review of our two years at County. The tone changed, we were set free, and we moved forward with gaiety. Now came the diplomas. As each graduate's name was called he or she went forward to the podium to accept their diploma. Individual groups went wild as their son, daughter, mother, wife, or lover took hold of a parchment tied with blue ribbon, and waved it in the air.

My turn came, and I wondered, would they be quiet and dignified, or would they scream like banshees. The event called for banshees, and my family let loose with their best. Jeff crowded the foot of the stage. He had his Nikon, his infinity lens, his flash; he looked like he was from the L.A. Times. I was embarrassed. I felt silly, and I also thought it was super sweet. In the flash of a strobe, my moment passed. It was time to move on, and let another assume the spot light. We sat in our chairs and waited, yelling and screaming, as each of our friends received their degree. We had released completely with dignity. This was a wild, happy celebration. Poor Madame President, she should have given up, and let us have the theme from "Bonanza" to march to.

A graduation ceremony is never the time to say anything meaningful to anyone. Everything is much too chaotic. Friends lose sight of one another as families gather around and gobble up their new graduates. We marched out of the doors, and into the arms of those who had loved us and supported us from behind the scenes. They hadn't fought the battles with us, but their love had been enduring. I think we were all happy to leave the battle behind. We were ready to join the outside world of our families and friends once again.

I lost sight of them all. Every one of my nursing friends was swept away into a sea of people who had come to claim them, just as I was. Jeff hugged me, kissed me, and began taking more pictures. My clan gathered around me, embraced me, and generally began celebrating the wonder of me. My father as usual was checking out my attire. "That's a great looking outfit. I hope you're going to wear it out to lunch, especially the hat."

"No Father, I can't be seen anywhere in public in this getup. I have to change at Jeff's. We'll meet you at the restaurant." My father was really disappointed; the man is mad for hats. From that point on, my memories of graduation turn into a white blur of stockings, shoes, a crumpled dress, and a stiff white cap, with a black velvet ribbon, left in a pile on the floor. All things to be sorted out later.

the end

Afterward

County gave their graduating seniors two months after graduation to find other housing, and to move. I thought this was exceptionally decent of them. One by one, we drifted off, and so the leaving had no clear closure. Little by little, we released our claim on the dorm. We withdrew our unique energies, to let the newcomers infuse it with their own.

All of my friends, myself included, passed our state boards on the first try. Sam, of course, moved to the West side. He became a surgical nurse, and worked at County for a while. He was absolutely right, our lives took such different turns, we let our friendship slide away. It was a mutual decision, and one I have always regretted.

Immediately upon graduation I went to work on 6A, the adolescent psychiatric unit. I became a member of the family there and Annie Sherman claimed me as her daughter. She has retired now and can frequently be found cruising on the Love Boat. Eighteen months after graduation I found I needed a break from County. Evelyn, Susan and I all end up working for the Red Cross, drawing blood from donors. It was a great job and a wonderful change from County. I converted Evelyn to the joys of Pasadena, and for several years we both lived there. Evelyn and I remain good friends; she keeps me updated on the progress of her two beautiful sons. Susan and I kept in touch for a short while. The last time all three of us were together was two years after graduation. We had dinner at Evelyn's house. We talked about life, and men, and women. I told them I was breaking up with Jeff and moving into my own apartment. I was surprised that my friends and family all greeted this news with a sigh of relief. Our dinner lasted late into the evening. I remember thinking how wonderful my friends looked in the glow of the candle light. I think this was the last time either Evelyn or I saw Susan. She was always elusive; Susan slipped away from us like a butterfly.

On a whim, and a moments notice, I enrolled myself in a Chiropractic College. After four years I required my family to attend yet another ceremony celebrating my becoming a Doctor of Chiropractic. A year later I treated myself to a horseback ride through France where I met the man I had been looking for all of my life. Fortunately, Larry had also been looking for me. We were married in Hawaii. Our maltese dogs Charlotte and Maggie May, along with my horse Shilo, round out our family.

I began this book because my time at County mystified me. I wondered why I had been so determined to place myself in that experience. I have now walked myself through those two years again. I have gone back to the smells, the sights, the work, and most importantly the people. I have let myself see retrospectively what I didn't see then. I have held my heart open through the process, to let the experiences flow through me once again. And, like the other difficult experiences in my life, this has been a gift to me.

I am not exactly the same person I was ten years ago. I have continued to evolve and change. It is not easy to look on the young woman I was at County, and at times, not to feel frustration or regret. I have wished at moments, that I could have shaken her, and told her to pay more attention; to tread more gently with others and herself. County gave me a chance to learn about myself, to explode some of the myths I have carried of my limitations. I had chosen County because I knew it would be hellacious. I was right. Some wonderful inner source told me it was time, time to move past old fears and limitations, to face mental monsters, and to stop allowing them to define my world.

Writing has given me a chance to watch myself in action. I have seen me wielding a heavy sword, and eyes closed, charge my dragons. I have given myself the opportunity to take another look, and this time to look beneath the surface. I wanted to explore the lessons of the time, so they wouldn't slip away from me unnoted. County for me was a portal; to be entered, participated in and passed through. Each time I walk through an archway, I find the opening on the other side is larger. It is a good thing, for there is always more of me to come out.

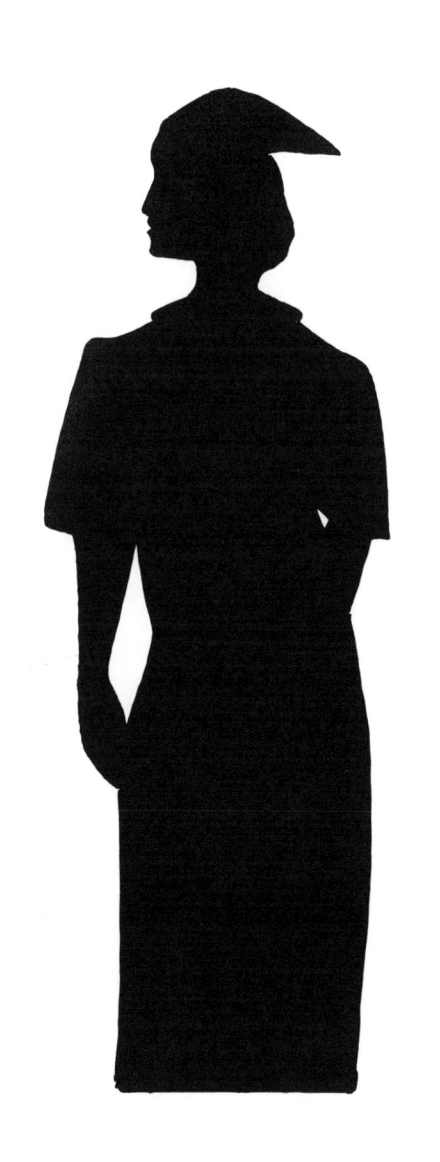